Pearls for your Practice

Pearls

for your

Practice

Dr. Joe Blaes

Copyright © 2001 by
PennWell Corporation
1421 South Sheridan Road
Post Office Box 1260
Tulsa, OK 74112-6600

800-752-9764
sales@pennwell.com
www.pennwell-store.com
www.pennwell.com

Cover and design by Robin Brumley

Library of Congress Cataloging-in-Publication Data

Blaes, Joseph A., DDS
    Pearls for Your Practice
    Joseph A. Blaes, DDS
        p. cm.
        q.cm
    Includes index
    ISBN 0-87814-820-5

Printed in the United States of America

1 2 3 4 5   05 04 03 02 01

Table of Contents

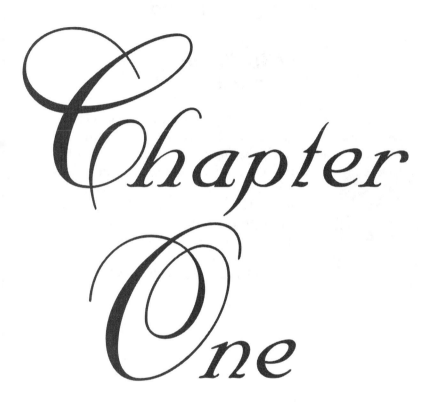

Chapter One

Materials, Equipment and Supplies

● ●

Pearl One

The IBC Brush
by Ultradent

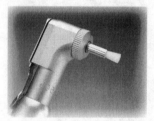

T his is a must-have item for every treatment room, including hygiene. I use these tiny brushes for every imaginable procedure that requires some form of polishing. They are great for polishing close to the gingival, because they are soft and do not tend to damage the tissue and cause bleeding. The hygienist loves them for cleaning in all those hard-to-reach places like orthodontic brackets. The bristles spread out, clean well, and do not fall out or get droopy. To order, call Ultradent at (800) 552-5512.

Pearl Two

Microbrush
by Microbrush Corporation

In answer to your requests, my favorite applicator now comes in "Regular" and "Fine" sizes. The fine size is smaller in diameter, allowing you to get to those tiny areas that were difficult with the regular size. With this addition, there is absolutely no reason to still be using bristle brushes. Do you realize how much material you waste with bristle brushes? Microbrushes will allow you to actually wipe off excess material on or near gingival tissues without fear of causing bleeding. They are great for seating veneers and crowns. If you like the feeling of a long handle, the Microbrushes come as inserts for handles, and the han- 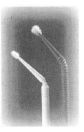 dles can be autoclaved. So throw out those awful bristle brushes and order some Microbrushes from your dealer! They come in a new packaging system with four colors. An even smaller brush is now available. I find more uses for them every day.

Pearl Three

Dry Tips
by Microscopy

A number of you have tried and are using the flat absorbent paper products to block the flow from the parotid gland. Although similar in appearance, Dry Tips actually are composed of three separate layers: (1) a nylon mesh fabric that gently adheres to the mucous-membrane, (2) the core, a polyacrylate/cellulose superabsorbent that retains moisture, and (3) a transparent polyethylene film moisture barrier on the outside toward the oral cavity. I have tried a few samples of the triangular paper products over the years, but always went back to the rubber dam or cotton rolls. But Dry Tips are different. Imagine work-

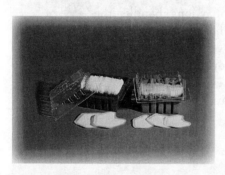

ing without concern of moisture contamination or the irritation of changing cotton rolls or absorbent pads in the middle of a difficult procedure. Dry Tips have many features including: (a) tremendous saliva absorption capacity; (b) even after becoming fully saturated, they can be handled without losing the absorbed moisture; (c) complete coverage of the parotid orifice and the entire buccal mucosa; (d) actually sticks to the mucous membrane and stays in place, yet it removes easily with no loose fibers or other residues left in the mouth; (e) protects the buccal mucosa and facilitates work far back in the oral cavity (makes those crown preps on the second molar much easier); (f) it's flexible, accommodates to cheek movements, and it comes in two sizes, adult and child. Dry Tips absorb and retain 30 times their own weight in moisture! This is a must-have item; they make sealants a snap. Order from Microcopy at (800) 235-1863. Try them once and you will be hooked like I am!

Pearl Four

Absorb-its and Safety Wipes
by Medical Innovations

When was the last time you had trouble keeping a cotton roll in place on the lingual of the lower anteriors? Absorb-its is a great new product to solve that problem and many more. The unique, anatomical shape is extremely comfortable for patients. The cellulose material effectively maintains a dry field, and it will not stick to the tissue. The softness allows them to be folded, twisted, or bent to creatively fit comfortably anywhere in the oral cavity. There is no need to buy different sizes. I have found Absorb-its to be great for doing bonding procedures on upper and lower anteriors. The Safety-wipes are meant to replace the 2" x 2" gauze wipe that the hygienist uses to clean instruments while scaling. Give both of these products a try by calling Medical Innovations at (800) 826-5650.

● ●

Pearl Five

Fitted Glove
by SS White

T he number-one area of musculoskeletal pain in a dentist's body occurs in his or her hands. Hand weakness is reported by one-third of all hygienists. Many profes-

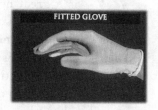

FITTED GLOVE

sionals whom I have observed do not wear gloves that fit properly. For many years, I have been wearing fitted gloves for all procedures. I have found that they are much, much more comfortable than ambidextrous exam gloves. The exam gloves tend to leave my hands fatigued and stressed. Fitted gloves allow proper blood supply to the muscles and allow you to work in a natural, relaxed position. An orthopedic surgeon would not consider the use of an ambidextrous exam glove. The SS White Fitted Glove will give you an extremely comfortable fit without baggy fingers, a great tactile sense so important in today's cosmetic procedures, and the ability to wear gloves for long periods of time. All of this at an affordable price—not much more than you would pay for exam gloves. These gloves are not just for the dentist; get some for your hygienists and assistants, too. If hand irritations are a concern, the SS White Ultimate PF is the only fitted glove that is powder-free. An ambidextrous fitted nitrite glove is also now available. SS White offers a no-risk guarantee, so what have you got to lose? Order from your dealer or call SS White at (800) 535-2877 for samples.

Pearl Six

Biogel Gloves
by Regent Medical

I discovered when I first began wearing gloves that I have less finger fatigue and a better fit and feel if I wear sized right/left gloves. Now Regent, the world leader in medical gloves, brings a powder-free, sized glove to dentistry to eliminate starch glove powder complications. The Biogel brand is the world's finest surgical glove with a Biogel coating for easy donning with wet or dry hands. The gloves offer a curved finger design for out-

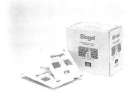

standing comfort, fit, and feel, and they come with a beaded cuff to reduce roll-down. They are packaged sterile and are available in right/left in half-sizes from 5-1/2 to 9. Regent makes a number of other styles of right/left gloves. As you might expect, these gloves are more expensive than what you are using now, but they are extremely comfortable for those long procedures and are much more durable. Call Regent Medical at (888) 566-3662 for more information, for samples, or to order.

Pearl Seven

DASH Gloves
by DASH Medical Gloves

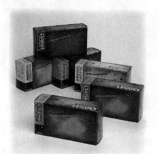

This latex-glove manufacturer is doing something about the allergies that many health-care workers experience. New processing dramatically reduces chemical irritants and lowers the latex protein. DASH offers powder-free latex gloves, lightly powdered latex gloves, and a latex-free synthetic glove. They offer a broad range of glove sizes for a comfortable fit. My hygienist was having some skin-rash problems and switched to these gloves. Her rash has since cleared up and has not reappeared. If you are having problems, try this line of gloves. Call DASH at (800) 523-2055 for samples or to order.

$\mathscr{P}earl$ $\mathscr{E}ight$

The 1838 Mask
by 3M Dental Products

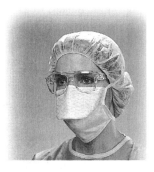

I have always felt that if we are going to wear a face mask for dental procedures, we should wear one that really protects. Through the years, I have searched and tried all of the dental masks on the market. I finally found one that is comfortable with a very high protection level. The only problem you will encounter is access to the product. The dental mask by 3M is a model 1818, but it is not the same. The 1838 mask must be purchased from a medical supply house since dental dealers do not carry this model. It is a tie-on mask that fits the face extremely well (no gapping holes!) and has a "duckbill" design that prevents the mask from touching the nose and mouth. It is great for long procedures because it is so comfortable. To place your order or to obtain additional information on the 3M 1838 Mask, contact your local medical supply company.

$\mathcal{P}earl\ \mathcal{N}ine$

Steri-Tip
by Great White, Inc.

I came across this very innovative, well-designed air/water syringe tip at the Greater New York Dental Meeting. Using an adapter supplied by Steri-Tip, these tips are quick and easy to place on the syringe. The innovative adapter design allows for a variable spray— 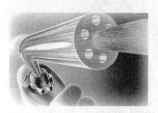 from a superfine mist to a coarse spray. There is no leaking, and they are strong enough to retract the cheek. Because of the design of the adapter and tip, very little maintenance is necessary. The low-cost tips help reduce overhead. Patients are very concerned about dental office cleanliness, and they expect us to use disposable items whenever possible. These tips were designed and are being marketed by two dentists. Call (973) 633-5963.

Pearl Ten

Nonlatex Dental Dam
by Hygienic

I have not had it happen in my office as yet, but I have heard lots of stories of patients' latex allergies. One precaution that I always recommend is the use of a rubber dam napkin to keep the latex off the face. We have recently tried a new nonlatex dam product from Hygienic that works adequately as a substitute. It is hard to compare it to latex because it is not latex. It does not seem to stretch as much, but it did the job. I would recommend giving it a try and having some on hand for that potential allergy patient. Order from your dealer.

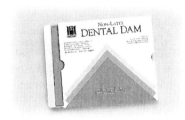

Pearl Eleven

Roto-Vac®
by Young Dental

I have been using the Roto-Vac® for years. My dental assistants love it because it is so simple to aspirate with. Most dental assistants have been taught to use a "palm thumb grasp" to hold a regular aspirating tip. They must get into some crazy positions to get the tip where the dentist wants it, and then they continually fight the hose. The Roto-Vac® eliminates all of this because you hold it in a "pen grasp"

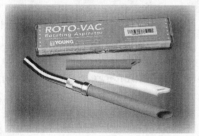

and then simply rotate the tip where you want it to go. The tip will rotate 360° and is made of stainless steel that will last a lifetime. A removable, disposable plastic tip slides over the patient end of the tip. After learning how to use the Roto-Vac® aspirating tip, your assistant will have less stress and fatigue at the dental chair. Order from your dealer. Don't accept any substitutes—insist on the Roto-Vac® from Young Dental.

$\mathscr{P}earl$ $\mathscr{T}welve$

Evacuation-System Maintenance
by Palmero Health Care

Have you ever wondered how effective some of the cleaning solutions are that you run through your evacuation systems? I often have wondered if they really did any good. Leave it to Ken Palmero to come up with two products that will keep your evacuation system sparkling clean. Shock 'ta' Clear is a pre-cleaning tablet that will strip the system clean of built-up bioburden. You use the Shock tablets on your system first. The next step is to use Vac-K 'ta' Clear tablets. You simply place these tablets in the chairside solids collector. This is a time-released tablet that will last for five days. Each time liquid passes over this tablet, cleaning chemicals are released into the system's lines. This product contains 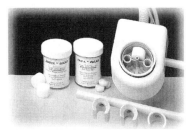 quaternary ammonium, which is a known antimicrobial and cleaning agent. It is guaranteed by the manufacturer to be 100 percent effective. Call Palmero Health Care at (800) 344-6424 for more information.

● ●

Pearl Thirteen

OralCDx®
by Sullivan-Schein Dental

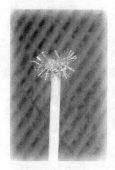

Oral cancer kills more people nationwide than skin cancer or cervical cancer. Recent studies show that benign-appearing, but potentially dangerous, oral lesions appear in 5 to 15 percent of the patients we see. Now for the first time, a tool takes the guesswork out of identifying the oral lesions that need further attention. You will never have to guess about the significance of an oral lesion again. OralCDx® is a computer-assisted, brush biopsy test for the detection of oral cancer. Now we have a rapid chairside procedure (similar to a pap smear) that requires no topical or local anesthetic. In the United States, a multicenter clinical trial of almost 1,000 patients was conducted at 35 academic dental centers. The outcome showed the OralCDx® test to be very precise. OralCDx® uncovered precancer or cancer among clinically benign-appearing lesions that would not have received additional testing or attention other than clinical follow-up, and which were judged harmless in appearance by experienced academicians. The complete study was published as the cover story in the October issue of JADA. This test is an extremely important benefit for your patients and another value-added benefit for your practice. There are two additional fees for the patient, one for the brush biopsy procedure that you performed and the second for the laboratory analysis. Both fees are reimbursed by the patient's medical or dental insurance. You file a claim for the in-office procedure, and the OralScan Laboratory submits a claim for the lab analysis. The test kits are provided free of charge by Sullivan-Schein Dental. Call (800) 560-4467 for an introductory package that contains an instructional video and five test kits. For more information, contact your Sullivan-Schein Dental representative or visit www.oral-cdx.com. Don't procrastinate on this one—early detection could save a life in your practice.

$\mathcal{P}earl$ $\mathcal{F}ourteen$

Yashica Dental Eye III
by Yashica Corporation

I have been using the Yashica Dental Eye since it first became available as the Dental Eye I years ago. If clinical photography is important to you, and you want a camera that you and your staff can easily pick up, turn on, and operate, this one's for you! We were amazed, because there was no learning curve to this camera. We unpacked it and imme- diately began shooting great slides. How many times have you left your camera on and put it away? The next time you use it there is no power because the batteries are dead. Not with this 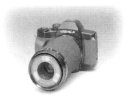 one! The power turns off in 30 seconds when no camera controls are used in order to conserve battery power. This camera is designed to give you the highest-quality photographs without a lot of complicated adjustments. The camera features auto film load and auto film advance, which helps when you are shooting a technique for a presentation. The Dental Eye III has a 100 mm macro lens and a built-in advanced flash system that results in much more detailed images. An LCD panel displays film counter and battery status. The viewfinder has been engineered to be brighter for eas- ier focusing—a real plus. The automatic film rewinder operates at high speed, so there is no time wasted between loading rolls. It has a flash hot shoe that enables you to attach an optional external flash. The camera has a smaller, lighter body with an ergonomic rubberized grip, which makes it easy to hold without movement. Customer service is great! I once had a problem with my Dental Eye I. I sent the camera back, and they fixed it and returned it to me in less than a week. Call Yashica Corporation at (800) 526-0266.

$\mathcal{P}earl$ $\mathcal{F}ifteen$

Macro 5 SLR Camera
by Polaroid Healthcare

I maging. I am sure that many of you already own this wonderful camera. I just got mine a few weeks ago and already I am in love with it! This simple camera makes it quick and easy to get the clear images

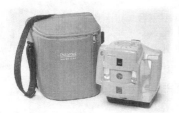

you need. Fully automatic and simple to operate, the lightweight Macro 5 has five built-in precision lenses. You simply turn the dial on top of the camera to choose the magnification you desire, from 20 to 300 percent. The Single Lens Reflex ensures that what you see is exactly what you photograph.

The magic of this camera is the "Light Lock" focusing system. You simply move the camera in and out until the two easy-to-see beams of light intersect, and the camera is in perfect focus. Then take your photograph. With the Macro 5, you can immediately and clearly show patients the work you have done and how it has improved their appearance.

These clear, precise pre- and post-treatment images also can be a powerful way to market your successes to new and existing patients. Many dentists have found that including photos along with claim forms can cut reimbursement time in half. The high-resolution, instant images also can be used for supplementing dental charts, giving the lab more information on the case and showing shade and changes from bleaching.

I use a technique that I learned from Dr. Mark Friedman, a great cosmetic dentist from San Diego. When he finishes a cosmetic case, he does not give patients a mirror. Instead, he takes an instant "after" picture to match patients' "before" picture. He then has his patient get out of the chair and stand before a mirror to look at the finished case. Along the border of the mirror, Dr. Friedman attaches the "before and after" pictures to remind patients how they looked and to give them a close-up look at the finished case. I am using this technique with great success.

The cost is a surprise, too. You can have this amazing, foolproof camera for under $750. Even better, the Macro 5 comes with a 30-day money-back guarantee, so you can try it risk-free. If you are doing any cosmetic dentistry, you must have this camera. Call (800) 315-0478, Ext. 11A, or visit www.polaroid.com/healthcare.

Pearl Sixteen

Intraoral Camera Mirror Attachment
by Polaroid

This is an FYI for those who have bought the Polaroid Macro 5 SLR or Polaroid Macro 3 SLR cameras. Polaroid now offers an Intraoral Dental Photography kit that retrofits these cameras, making them even more valuable in the dental treatment room. The mirrors attach to the front of the cameras so you can take perfect photos without anyone's help. The Polaroid Macro 5 SLR was a great camera before now, but with the addition of the mirrors, it is an excellent

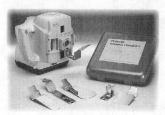

camera. If you want to enhance your cosmetic practice, call Polaroid immediately at (800) 662-8337, ext. H012, and find out where to buy one of these cameras! Or just call Photomed at (800) 998-7765 and they will ship one right out to you.

Pearl Seventeen

LH Systems Cleaner
by Nu Source International

Now comes help for the most unpopular job in the office — cleaning the X-ray processor or the manual tanks in the darkroom. Nu Source has introduced LH, a Low Hazard systems cleaner. This is a one-part, fast-acting, concentrated powder cleaner designed to speedily dissolve silver oxide deposits and other stains from developer and fixer tanks and roller assemblies in automatic processors and manual tanks. It will not harm rubber rollers even with extended soaking. The material is personally and environmentally safe to use, and it requires no hazardous duty fee when shipping or receiving. Nu Source also provides easy-to-use and environmentally safe developers and fixers, which feature the latest advancements in darkroom-chemical technology. Whether your needs are for automatic, manual, and endo/rapid applications, or fast-acting, low-hazard, powdered systems cleaners, a full line of products helps minimize risks associated with chemicals in the darkroom. Fixscent, a specially formulated deodorizer, completely eliminates chemical odors and provides a fresh, pleasant, floral fragrance. Color Check, a unique color-coding system, helps eliminate possible cross-contamination. If minimal cross-contamination occurs when using the Red developer and the Blue fixer, the contaminated product will become clear, thus alerting the assistant that contamination has occurred. The new formulation has excellent resistance to oxidation, which means it works cleaner and has a longer active life. It will develop more films over a longer period, while maintaining high-quality images. Call Nu Source International at (815) 477-9844.

● ●

Pearl Eighteen

TTL Telescopes
by Orascoptic Research, Inc.

I have been using magnification for years now and would not think of picking up a handpiece without scopes. I believe that magnification is now the standard of care in dentistry. I have been using Designs for Vision magnifiers for years and putting up with poor customer service because I liked the glasses. Recently, I was introduced to the Orascoptic line of magnifiers. The Orascoptic TTL is a new line of 2.5x 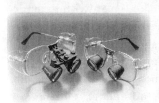 fixed-position, "through the lens" telescopes. This company, led by the founder and researcher, Dr. Charles Caplan, has developed telescopes that will enhance comfort, performance, and safety. These glasses are very comfortable to wear and provide high resolution optics with a wide depth and width-of-field. The nosepiece is particularly well done and provides a good base for the telescopes. I am convinced that magnifiers help me complete treatment faster, better and easier. These Orascoptic telescopes give me comfort and excellent visual clarity. Combined with the Zeon Illuminator, you have a team that cannot be beat. Orascoptic is introducing a new line of scopes for the rest of the dental team that will allow the assistants to actually see what they are doing. The hygienists also will benefit from this new line. Orascoptic provides excellent customer service and follow-up to assure that you are completely satisfied with the product. It is nice to know that someone out there cares. Call Orascoptic Research, Inc. at (800) 369-3698 to order, or stop by and see them at the Chicago Midwinter and get measured right at the booth.

Pearl Nineteen

The Zeon Illuminator
by Orascoptic Research, Inc.

I have tried most of the light sources that come with dental magnifiers and have found them all to be either rather cumbersome and uncomfortable or the light was not very good. So I was reluctant to try another one. I finally ordered one from Orascoptic, and, when it came in, I was on the road. My new partner opened the box and set it up. He immediately fell in love with the system. I had to wrestle it away from him to try it for myself. Dr. Mark was right. The Zeon system is great! It is a lightweight system that will fill not only

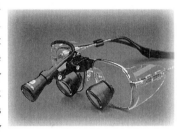

Orascoptic magnifiers, but other brands as well. So, if you already have magnification, you can add the Zeon Illuminator to it. There will be no more miner's helmets or heavy wires to contend with. The light is fantastic! I have prepped with the operating light with the fiber optics in the handpiece turned off and had better light than I ever experienced before. You will be amazed at what you can see. And this is brilliant, shadowless, line-of-sight illumination that frees you and your assistant of the frequent adjustments to the standard operatory light. Line of sight means that the light goes with you when you turn your head or look at an impression or temporary outside the mouth. Based on our experience with the system, I would recommend that you buy your handpieces without fiber optics and use the Zeon Illuminator instead. That is one less thing to go wrong with the handpiece. This is a no-brainer! Call Orascoptic Research, Inc. at (800) 369-3698 for more information.

$\mathcal{P}earl\ \mathcal{T}wenty$

Pearls
by Orascoptic Research, Inc.

I have always wondered why there was not a magnification line available to assistants and hygienists. After all, they need to see well too. Orascoptic is stepping in to fill that void with a line of magnifying glasses for your hygienist and your assistant. These truly unique 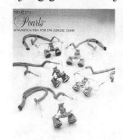 glasses are made from the ever-popular Gargoyles frame design, giving your auxiliaries that stylish feel. They are available in three working distances to provide comfortable, ergonomic posture and relieve common back, neck, and shoulder discomfort. A unique double-hinge system will adjust to your working angle and will enable oculars to be flipped up for unmagnified vision. The telescopes can be individually designed or Gargoyles can be made with interchangeable prescriptions for sharing. And they come in great colors as well. Call Orascoptic Research, Inc. at (800) 369-3698 to order.

Pearl Twenty-one

Improved Model of Zeon Illuminator
by Orascoptic Research, Inc.

Orascoptic has made some significant improvements in this illuminator system. The box that houses the light source is smaller and lighter, and it has a recessed handle for ease of movement. There are now dual intensity controls with an adjustable iris to control intensity while maintaining constant color temperature. The other intensity control adjusts the voltage intensity to increase the life of the bulb. The fiber-optic cable is lighter and easier to adapt to your magnifying glasses. Once you add this illuminator to your treatment room, you can forget about handpiece fiber optics. The bottom line is that you will see better, feel better, and perform better because you can 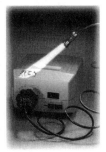 see better! Beware: Once you use this, you will never use any other light source! To order, call (800) 369-3698 or visit www.orascoptic.com.

Pearl Twenty-two

The Bora High-Speed Handpiece
by Bien Air

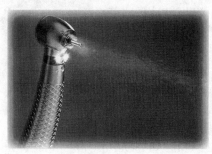

This is a Swiss handpiece company that you probably have not heard of before. But you should be aware of it because it makes excellent handpieces in all sizes and shapes. I was introduced to this handpiece at the California meeting in Anaheim in April and have been using it since then. I am very impressed. The handpiece has held up well after multiple sterilizations, and the push-button bur changer works well. The handpiece system comes with a quick-release coupling that allows it to rotate 360 degrees and is compatible with all the Bien Air motors. A new air hose system allows exhaust air to be channeled away from the patient and operator. The fiber optics is a double glass rod system that seems to be holding up well. Are you tired of replacing handpiece bearings? Then try the Bien Air GYRO air-bearing handpiece. This revolutionary handpiece does not have any bearings— nothing to wear out! The very first handpiece I had was an air-bearing by Encore. The firm went out of business, or I would still be using that handpiece. Bien Air has improved on the Encore design, providing a number of new advancements. It requires no greasing or any other kind of lubrication, so it is great for your cosmetic cases. It does require a learning curve on cutting with it, because you can stall it out easier, but that is not a great problem. Take a look at this one—think of all the time and money you would save on bearing replacements! Bien Air also has a great electric handpiece that we are just beginning to look at—more on that later. This is a solid company with many innovative products. Be sure to check it out. For more information, call Bien Air at (800) 433-BIEN.

Pearl Twenty-three

Prismatic Loupes
by Orascoptic Research, Inc.

N ow, we have more power from the folks at Orascoptic. These loupes are available in 3.8 times, 4.3 times, and 4.8 times magnification. They are the TTL ("through-the-lens") type of loupes designed to provide a large field, bright optics, and exceptional resolution. The frames are made of titanium for strength and are lightweight. The high-powered lens has an adjustment that allows you to set the distance you like to work from perfectly. This is really great because you don't have to move your body back and forth to find the working distance set for the glasses. In the past, if the 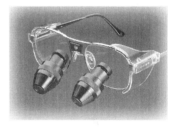 person measuring you for the magnifiers did not measure the working distance correctly, then you had some stress problems moving your body into position. The loupes are lightweight and do not seem heavy on the nose. The magnification is fantastic. Now, you can really see the margins on those crown preps! The Zeon Illuminator fits these loupes and provides great lighting exactly where you need it. I do not use fiber-optic handpieces any longer because the lighting is so much better with the Zeon. If you are in the market for magnification (and you should be if you don't have any), then go see the folks at Orascoptic. You can try the glass risk-free—what have you got to lose? Call them at (800) 369-3698 today!

Pearl Twenty-four

KaVo 640B and 642B Handpieces
by KaVo America

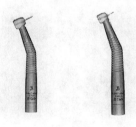

As I lecture at various meetings around the country, I usually am challenged because I have not tried the KaVo Handpiece. So, for the last eight months, I have been using two KaVo high-speed handpieces-the 640B and the 642B. I have used them on a regular basis and found them to be superior handpieces that are very quiet during operation. These are very high torque handpieces, yet extremely smooth with virtually no vibration. The handpiece comes with a 360-degree swivel that gets rid of the bothersome drag from the tubing. The 640B standard head with its outstanding torque is designed for crown and bridge work and bulk removal. Its three-port spray cooling gets the water to the tooth for cooling and dentin removal. The 642B miniature head is excellent for pedo work in areas with difficult access. The unique cellular optic lighting system on both handpieces is one of the best that I have seen, and it provides good, bright, color-corrected light to the teeth you are working on. These cellular optics won't break down after sterilization. KaVo guarantees that with a five-year warranty on its cellular optics. With the Multiflex coupler system, it is very easy to connect to every five-hole fiber-optic or six-hole power optic tubing. It is very easy to change handpieces with this system due to a great quick-disconnect that has an anti-retraction valve. The burs are changed with an auto chuck, making that chore fast and easy with no bur slippage, and they run concentric. The handpieces have been in daily usage and have been sterilized many times without any problems. KaVo America is known as a company that stands behind its products and is interested in providing excellent customer service. So order your KaVo handpiece from your dealer today, or call KaVo America at (888) KaVo USA (888-528-6872) to get more information or answers to your questions.

Pearl Twenty-five

The 430 Series High-Speed Handpieces
by Star Dental

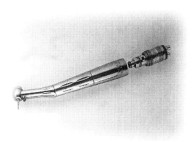

I have been using the Star 430 high-speed handpiece since 1977, when I purchased eight of the 430 SWL handpieces. These handpieces are still in daily service today. Over the years, Star has been an innovator in handpiece design, and always has stood behind its products. Now, the company has done it again with a new 430 handpiece. Star now employs a unique Vortex Air Seal Design that seals the turbine from debris spiraling up the bur shaft. Drive air leakage through the front bearing also is blocked, preventing the escape of lubricants or other contaminants that reduce the bond strength of restorations. Today's heat sterilization places high demands on conventional high-speed handpieces. The 430 Series exceeds expectations by offering greater durability to accommodate today's high number of autoclave/chemiclave cycles. That's why the 430 Series handpiece—with its exclusive lube-free turbine and vortex air seal design; longer-lasting fiber optics; protective, medical-grade coating; and dependable cutting power—merits the industry's best and longest hassle-free warranty. If you are in the market for new handpieces, take a good look at the Star 430 Series. I think you will be very happy with it.

● ●

Pearl Twenty-six

The Electric Micromotor Handpiece
by Bien Air

Wow! What a handpiece! I cannot believe the torque of this new handpiece from Bien Air. This is an electric micromotor-driven handpiece that will accept a number of different speed handpieces. I have used the high-speed handpiece to prepare hundreds of crowns and would not use anything else to cut teeth. It

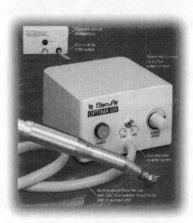

cuts quickly through porcelain and nonprecious metal with incredible torque. Enamel cuts quickly away. Crowns preps are quick and simple. The system is very quiet—the high-pitched air rotor scream is gone. Patients don't miss that scream at all! They are even more pleased by the absence of vibration from the handpiece and bur. I prepped 10 crowns the other day in record time without the usual hand fatigue. The speed range is great—from very slow for fine, precise work to fast for bulk reduction—all with no loss of torque. The control box can be quickly retrofitted to your unit so that you can use your regular foot control and water supply. This is one you need to see to believe. Bien Air is a Swiss-based company with offices around the world. They are the number-two dental handpiece seller in the world. Order from your dealer or call (800) 433-BIEN for more information.

$\mathscr{P}earl \quad \mathscr{T}wenty\text{-}seven$

RotoMix
by 3M ESPE

T raditionally, 3M ESPE has been the company to do innovative things with materials in capsules. I have used many of their products over the years. These mixers are designed especially for mixing the material capsule products for which they are famous. This is a unique design that will rotate the capsule instead of shaking it, and then spin it like a centrifuge. In the rotational cycle, the capsule spins counterdirectionally to the rotating platform. The material is mixed in all directions during this cycle to assure a completely homogeneous mix. In the centrifugal cycle, RotoMix locks the capsule in place on the rotating platform so that it spins with the platform. This step forces out any entrapped air so there are no air bubbles in the material. This step also allows the material to be dispensed far more easily. This is a significant step in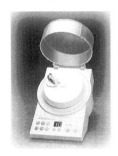
mixing materials. Capsulated dental materials were developed to facilitate higher powder-liquid ratios and a more consistent mix. How thoroughly the materials are mixed is significant to the final physical properties of the set material. The disadvantage of conventional mixers is the high amount of air that is incorporated into the material during the mix. I like the capsule idea for consistent mixes every time, and now I have a great new mixer to make them even more consistent. Order from your dealer or call 3M ESPE at (800) 344-8235.

Pearl Twenty-eight

Chemiclave Sterilizer
by Harvey

I have been sterilizing instruments without steam for so many years that I had forgotten about all the drawbacks of steam. There is no better way to extend the life of your instruments than not to use steam. The Harvey Chemiclave is a fully automated, proven device for sterilizing dental instruments without dulling, corroding, or otherwise impairing their properties. The shanks of your diamonds and burs will not rust like they do with steam. Your instruments come out bright and

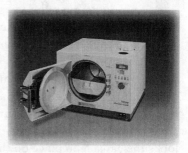

shiny with no hint of rust or corrosion. No more soggy bags. The chemical vapor process protects your investment in instruments and significantly reduces deterioration from corrosion. The cutting edges of your instruments will stay sharper longer. Your hygienist will love you! Because nothing ever gets wet, you do not need a time-consuming drying phase, and the Harvey Chemiclave is actually faster than conventional steam. Once you try this system and see the results, you will wonder why you put up with steam all these years. Order from your dealer or call Harvey at (800) 553-0039 for more information.

$\mathcal{P}earl$ $\mathcal{T}wenty$-nine

Gendex GX-LC
by Dentsply

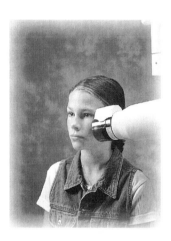

If you own a Gendex GX-770 X-ray, you will want to check out this new optically assisted positioning system. This is a lighted cone that uses a pinpoint of light to take the guesswork out of positioning the cone in relation to the film. The result is consistent, high-quality radiographic images. For additional information, call Gendex at (800) 800-2888 or contact your dealer.

● ● ● ● ● ● ● ● ● ● ● ● ● ● ● ● ● ● ● ●

Pearl Thirty

EzeeKleen 2.5
by Oasis Dental Group

This device is an alternative to distilled water. If you buy bottled, distilled water for your autoclave or have your own still, you need to look at this device. The EzeeKleen 2.5 is the way to manufacture quality water for your sterilizers quickly and easily. It will manufacture 4 liters of autoclave-safe water in approximately four minutes.

You will never again run out of water for the sterilizer. Stop those last-minute runs to the grocery store to replenish the distilled water. You will have no more storage problems, and you can monitor the quality of the water you produce. This unit utilizes a unique cartridge system to produce water that meets or exceeds autoclave-manufacturer requirements at a lower cost than anything you currently use.

It is easy to install and can be wall-mounted or counter-mounted. All components are quick-connected so that the cartridge changes take only seconds. Call Oasis Dental Group at (800) 338-6693.

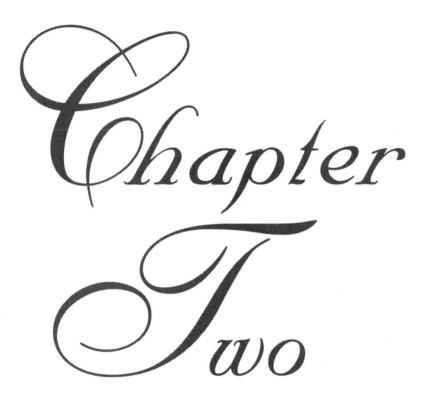

Chapter Two

Instruments

● ●

Pearl Thirty-one

DuraLite Instruments
by Nordent

I recently came across these instruments made by a company that has been around for more than 25 years in Chicago. Somehow, I had never heard of them. I am sure that some of you probably know of the company and love their instruments. The DuraLite is a lightweight handle designed for all your favorite instruments. The han-

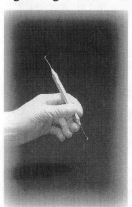

dle is ergonomically designed to rest comfortably in your hand, and this is exactly what it does. This instrument really does all that it claims. There is an incredible weight difference between our standard instrument pack and the pack with our new DuraLite instruments. Now, here is more good stuff: The handles are all stainless steel and are all handcrafted. They won't crack, peel, stain, or wear out—no matter what sterilization method you use. The handles have a light texturing that minimizes slipping. They are easy to clean because there are no deep grooves to trap tissue, blood, and debris. Because of the design, it will not roll around on the tray or roll off the tray onto the floor. Nordent has thought of everything, because it even fits in all cassette configurations. Whether you need diagnostic, hygiene, operative, or surgical instruments, take a look at Nordent for fine quality at a good value. My hygienist has tried the hygiene instruments and loves the feel and the lightness. She claims to have less hand fatigue at the end of the day. Take a look at this great line of instruments. They are guaranteed! Call Nordent at (800) 966-7336.

Pearl Thirty-two

Zekrya Gingival Retractor and Protector
by Zenith Dental Products

If you do any procedures close to the gingival tissue, you need this instrument. I don't know how I ever practiced without it! It has made almost every procedure I do easier and less traumatic for the patient. Just think of all the times you could have used an instrument that not only gently retracts the tissue, but also protects the tissue from burs, diamonds, and excavators. This is the one. Use it to retract and/or protect tissue for veneer preps, finishing veneer margins, checking marginal fit of crowns, Class V preps, Class V subgingival caries removal, and checking for loose crowns or bridges. The Zekrya prevents bleeding—no more blood to interfere with cementation of a veneer or the polymerization of a composite. Now you can see your margins!

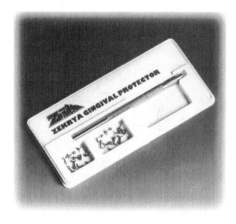

You can refine the margin and place it exactly where you want it. No more guessing! The Zekrya has a swivel joint, which allows for a simple adjustment to reach any desired position. There is a wide and narrow arc that allows for adaptation to all size teeth. The protector arcs can be reused and autoclaved, so they are cost-effective. When the arcs become scratched or marred, they are replaceable. It controls bleeding without chemicals and protects the tissue from being cut. This one is a no-brainer! If you want more accurate and controlled preparations, more accurate margins, and better dentistry easier than ever before, buy the Zekrya Gingival Protector. Order from your dealer.

Pearl Thirty-three

SuperMat Retainerless Matrix System
by Premier Dental Products Company

Placing and adjusting all matrix bands is now easier and more convenient than ever. Clear or metal bands are easily placed with the unique SuperMat instrument. The system consists of a placement instrument that is used in conjunction with the disposable spools to anchor and tighten the matrix band into the desired position. The

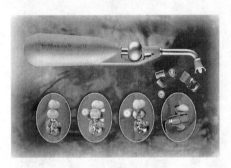

SuperMat spool secures the matrix band for a good gingival seal and ideal proximal contacts. The tension of the band can be increased or decreased easily at any time during the procedure. Since only the tiny SuperMat spool remains in the mouth, you have much easier access for wedging and for placement of the restorative material. Proper proximal contacts are easier to establish, because the traditional matrix retainer is not in your way. The SuperMat system improves your visibility, and your patient is much more comfortable since no retainer is needed. It also eliminates band movement or distortion due to the patient's lip movement. It can be used in conjunction with rubber dam or other isolation techniques. With this unique applicator system, several restorations can easily be completed simultaneously in the same quadrant. The SuperMat placement instrument can be autoclaved repeatedly, and no special instrument is required for removal of the matrix bands. This system is a great timesaver and will make your inventory of matrix bands much simpler. Remember, time is money! Order the SuperMat Retainerless Matrix System from your dealer.

$\mathcal{P}$earl $\mathcal{T}$hirty-four

The Craniometer
by Craniometrics, Inc.

One of the biggest problems in fixed and removable prostho-
dontics is the determination of the correct vertical dimension.
There are many methods for this determination, but all involve
some guesswork and some trial-and-error methods. Dr. Stanley
Knebelman, a general practitioner from Philadelphia, has invented a
wonderful instrument that will
eliminate the guesswork and
allow you to accurately determine
how much vertical dimension has
been lost. The Craniometer is
easy to use and comes with a
complete instructional video. The
distance between the external
auditory meatus and the lateral
border of the ocular orbit is meas-

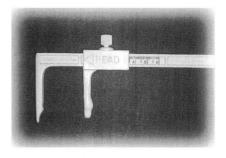

ured, recorded, and then the gauge is reset to the craniometric adjustment. When growth and development and occlusion are normal, the
gauge should fit snugly between the most anterior part of the under-
surface of the mandible and the nasal spine when the teeth are occlud-
ed. If it fits loosely, then there is a loss of occlusal vertical dimension.
You can easily restore back to the proper vertical. The Craniometer can
be used with natural teeth and with full denture cases. I have had great
success with this simple device. For more information or to order, call
(610) 642-4042. A training video is available.

Pearl Thirty-five

The Tri Auto-ZX
by J. Morita

Imagine an endodontic handpiece that also will locate the apex. Then imagine that it is cordless, and you have the Tri Auto-ZX from the people who brought you the highly suc- cessful and accurate Root-ZX apex finder. This low- speed endodontic handpiece, when combined with the Root-ZX, enables the clinician to monitor the root canal electronically before, during, and after instru- mentation. This handpiece has three automatic func- tions that are significant improvements and which eliminate the need for a foot control. First, the hand- piece automatically starts when the file enters the 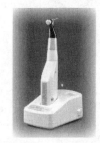 canal and stops when the file is removed. Second, the handpiece auto- matically stops and reverses the rotation of the nickel titanium file when too much pressure is applied. And third, the handpiece automat- ically stops and reverses the rotation of the file when the tip reaches a distance from the apex that has been preset by the clinician. An LED control panel on the handpiece monitors the position of the file tip dur- ing root-canal shaping and cleaning. The handpiece will shut off auto- matically after three minutes if not in use to conserve battery power. Call J. Morita at (800) 752-9729 for more details.

Pearl Thirty-six

Endo Analyzer 8005
by Analytic

I get excited when a dental manufacturer combines two functions in one instrument. The Endo Analyzer does exactly that. It combines state-of-the-art pulp testing and apex location in a single compact unit. I was listening to Dr. Cliff Ruddle present an endo seminar last week, and he stated that apex locators are 95 percent accurate. To me, that means that everyone who is doing endo should have one of these. This tool features a backlit screen with large numerical, as well as graphical, read-outs to give you precise information quickly and easily. The vitality scanning function is pain-free and automatically con- 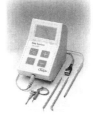 trolled for consistent testing. For additional information on the Endo Analyzer or to place your order, call Analytic at (800) 346-ENDO or visit their Web site at www.Analytic-Endodontics.com.

Pearl Thirty-seven

XCP Film Holder
by Dentsply Rinn

I have been using the XCP instrument for at least 25 years. My mentor, Dr. Roy Wolff, was a pedodontist who put me on to the technique when it first came out, and I have been using it ever since. You just don't miss using the XCP! No cone-cutting. No wrong angulations to cause distortion. It makes the paralleling technique a snap. Great X-rays, fast and simple, every time. After all these years, some great improvements in the system have been made. The transformation involves color-coding the film holder for easy assembly of the component parts. Assembly was always a problem, particularly while you were learning the system. Now there will be no more fumbling around trying to find the right combination to take that posterior film. All you have to do is match the colors. How come it took so long to figure that out?! The anterior film holder uses a blue bite block, blue pins on the arm, and a blue dot on the aiming ring. The posterior holder uses yellow coordinates. The bitewing film holder uses red coordinates. Dentsply Rinn has made the entire system fully autoclavable—a great step forward in infection control. They have also shortened the aiming arm to fit all intraoral X-ray units. Who says things don't get better with age? This is a no-brainer! Call your dealer and order an XCP film holder system for great images every time.

Pearl Thirty-eight

Profin Directional System
by Dentatus USA

I recently was reintroduced to the Profin System. Have you ever wished for a handpiece that would go back and forth instead of around? This unique attachment for your straight handpiece is the answer to your prayer. This instrument system moves some specially designed tips in a back-and-forth motion, rather than in the customary rotary action. I use the Profin System to gain access to the interproximal areas to remove amalgam overhangs. It works very well to remove and smooth resin when you are bonding cosmetic inlay. You always risk pitting or ditching when you use a rotary handpiece to do this procedure. The addition of many tips to the system has greatly enhanced the uses. The Profin System can be very useful in the finishing of all types of preparations. The addition of straight tips gives you a greater range of uses in removing all types of undercuts. This is the only handpiece system that I know of to safely finish the interproximal areas of the teeth. Try one; I know you will like it. Call Dentatus USA at (800) 323-3136 for more information or order from your dealer.

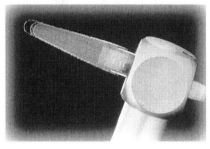

$\mathcal{P}earl$ $\mathcal{T}hirty\text{-}nine$

Expandex
by Parkell

T his is a great, inexpensive little instrument to hold the lips out of your way while doing procedures in the anterior part of the mouth. We use this compact lip retractor constantly, even underneath the

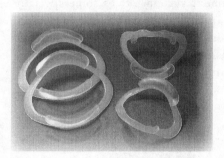

rubber dam. Expandex is a soft, flexible plastic frame that provides superb anterior isolation during any anterior procedure. The patient relaxes in comfort even if the procedure takes several hours. No more soggy cotton rolls. It comes in an adult version and a pediatric version. Call Parkell at (800) 243-7446 to order.

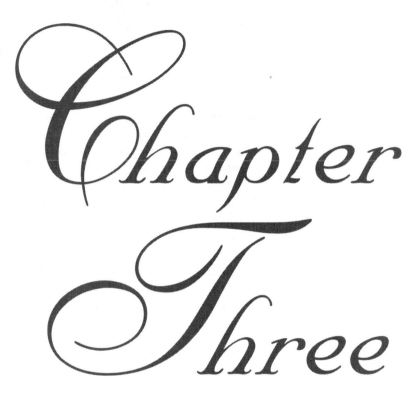

Chapter Three

Anesthesia

Pearl Forty

BD® Dental Needle
by Crosstex

BD(Becton Dickinson) makes most of the needles used in hospitals and physicians' offices. I first saw the BD Dental Needle at the Wisconsin State Meeting in May of 1999. As often happens these days, a good friend of mine said that he had a great product to

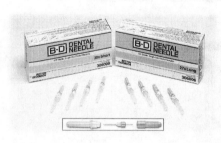

show me. At lunchtime, he literally dragged me onto the exhibit floor and over to a booth that was showing the new needle that he felt should be a pearl. At the booth, I looked at the needle and said, "So, someone else has entered the needle market; what's the big deal?" Well, BD has rigged up a "Sharpness Testing Device" that I tried, using my favorite needle as a comparison. The test was very convincing, so I decided I needed to try some of these needles on my patients. The next time you are at a meeting, stop by and try the test yourself. In the medical industry, BD is known for sharp needles. Sharp needles mean less pain when the needle penetrates tissue and less deflection of the needle as it moves through the tissue. I have found that the BD Dental Needle has a significant improvement in sharpness, and this results in dramatic reductions in both penetration and drag forces. What this means to patients is less pain and a quick, easy injection. For details, call Crosstex at (888) CROSSTEX (276-7783). Order from your dealer.

Pearl Forty-one

Palatal Anesthesia Device (PAD)
by Master Dental

This is a unique, simple instrument that will decrease greatly the pain associated with palatal injections. The instrument was developed by a practicing periodontist and uses the principles of pressure anesthesia and the gate-control theory of pain. Pressure anesthesia is administered by applying mechanical pressure with the C-shaped end of the instrument on the palatal tissue. The stimulation of the surface tactile receptors by the instrument "opens the gate" of the pain-transmitting fibers and interrupts their transmission to the brain. The pain of the initial needle penetration is reduced greatly. The C-shaped end is firmly pressed onto the palatal tissue until the tissue blanches. Then, the 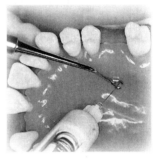 syringe needle is inserted gently into the palatal tissue through the open center of the C. Remove the instrument and slowly administer anesthetic. You have just given your most painless palatal injection, and your patient will never be afraid of palatal injections again. I could not believe that a technique this simple could be so very effective! This is one that you have to try. Call Master Dental at (517) 792-4431 for more information or to order.

● ● ● ● ● ● ● ● ● ● ● ● ● ● ● ● ● ● ●

Pearl Forty-two

DentiPatch
by Noven Pharmaceuticals, Inc.

This is a patch that is designed to be applied to the soft tissues of the mouth. It delivers profound Lidocaine anesthesia to the area to which it is applied, right to the depth of the bone. After application, you can penetrate to the bone with a 25-gauge needle, and the patient feels no pain. You now can confidently tell your phobic patients that you can get them numb without feeling a thing! There are a number of soft-tissue applications such as scaling and root planing, ultrasonic scaling, perio probe examination, and therapeutic fiber placement, all of which can be accomplished with complete comfort using the DentiPatch. Call Noven Pharmaceuticals, Inc., a leader in patch technology, at (888) 55-NOVEN.

● ● ● ● ● ●

Pearl Forty-three

Stabident
by Fairfax Dental

This is a local anesthesia system that I have been using for years. It is a totally new method of achieving local anesthesia by using intraosseous injection. It can be used as your primary system or as a back-up system when conventional methods fail. Stabident is simple to use, and patients remark that there is little postoperative discomfort from the injection site. The system involves using a handpiece-driven needle to perforate the cortical plate of bone, and then inserting an injector needle into that hole to deliver standard, local anesthetic to the cancellous bone. This causes deep, pulpal anesthesia immediately. You will be amazed at the results you can achieve on "hot" teeth. The Stabident system allows you to overcome one of the big problems in dentistry—inadequate anesthesia. Call Fairfax Dental today at (800) 233-2305 for more information. The company has an excellent demonstration video and instruction sheet that come with your first order.

Pearl Forty-four

Ultracare Topical Anesthetic
by Ultradent

I have been using Ultradent products since Dr. Dan Fischer introduced his first line of syringes and tips. I have been using Ultradent products for so long that I have forgotten to include them in "Pearls." The Ultracare topical anesthetic is one of these products. We

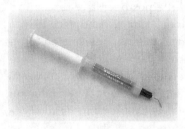

have used it as a topical before giving anesthesia. The combination of a pleasant taste and smell, rapid onset, and great effectiveness makes it the topical of choice in my office. But that is only one use of Ultracare! My hygienists would not practice without it, even though they are licensed to give local anesthetic in Missouri. The packaging is why they like it so much. Ultracare is packaged in single-dose 1.2cc syringes with White Mini tips that allow you to place the topical in and around the gingival sulcular tissues during root-planing and scaling procedures. It gives great anesthesia in a very specific area. My hygienists find that this is all they need to complete most procedures comfortably for the patient. It also eliminates all those Q-tips full of topical that usually are found in the hygiene treatment room after a periodontal-therapy procedure. The single-dose syringes also are great when a patient returns and needs only some site-specific therapy. You can put the topical right where you want it. Give Ultradent a call today at (800) 552-5512 and order some for your office.

$\mathscr{P}earl$ $\mathscr{F}orty\text{-}five$

The Wand
by Milestone Scientific

If you have been to a dental meeting since the ADA in Washington, you have seen the crowds around the booth showing The Wand. I must tell you that I was skeptical when I first saw The Wand at the ADA. Since then, I have become convinced that every dentist should have one. I would not want to receive anesthetic any other way. I know what you are thinking, because I thought the same thing: "I don't need a machine to give painless injections; I can do that myself." But you can't! The Wand is a computer-controlled, local-anesthesia delivery system. The Wand doesn't work like a syringe. A micro-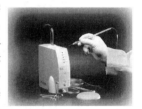processor delivers precise pressure and volume ratios of anesthetic. Even in resilient tissue, such as the palate and the periodontal ligament, The Wand maintains optimal flow for an effective, virtually pain-free injection. You begin the flow of anesthetic before needle insertion, so that an anesthetic drip precedes the needle. This "anesthetic pathway" means that there is virtually no sensation or pain as the needle penetrates to the target. All of this results in a pain-free injection and a rapid onset of profound anesthesia.

If you are doing any anterior esthetic dentistry, you must be using the new AMSA (Anterior Middle Superior Alveolar) nerve block. It allows you to anesthetize completely up to 10 maxillary teeth with only two needle penetrations and only one carpule of anesthetic. The Wand produces a suffusion of anesthetic solution into palatal tissue, yet always at a flow rate below the threshold of pain. You get profound pulpal anesthesia without anesthesia of the lip and facial muscles, so that smile-line considerations and assessments will not be hampered by facial distortion. This

● ●

reduces chair time and follow-up visits. The PDL (Periodontal Ligament Injection) is often avoided because it is difficult to administer, painful, and inconsistent. This new system's precision and control make PDL injections easier, more predictable, and completely comfortable. The Wand revolutionizes dental injections by taking away the fear and anxiety on the part of the patient and reducing stress for the dental team. Order from your dealer or call Milestone Scientific at (800) 862-1125.

Pearl Forty-six

X-tip Anesthesia Delivery System
by X-tip Technologies

L eave it to a couple of dentists to come up with the solution for "finding the hole!" The most frustrating problem with intraosseous anesthesia systems has always been to get the needle back into the hole that you have drilled in the bone. This problem

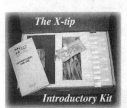

The X-tip

Introductory Kit

was the major reason I gave up on a great system for getting instant profound anesthesia. This system simply leaves a marker-the X-tip-where you drilled into the bone. I know you will find that this simple system will revolutionize your anesthesia technique. No more painful anterior injections, because placing an X-tip distal to the cuspid numbs all the teeth to the midline. Never again postpone treatment because you can't get a tooth numb! Don't even think about this one; pick up the phone and call (800) 215-4245 to order. If you are skeptical, order the Starter Kit for $29.95. I know you will be convinced and will shortly reorder a regular X-tip system!

Chapter Four

Bonding

Pearl Forty-seven

PermaQuick PQ1
by Ultradent

I have always been a fan of the syringe delivery systems for which Ultradent has become famous. PQ1 is a single-component bonding system that falls into that category as well. With a fast and easy syringe delivery system, all you need to do is add a tip to make this bonding agent the simplest to deliver. The delivery tip contains a small brush to aid in the precise delivery of the material. You get a strong bond with fluoride release. The material is 40 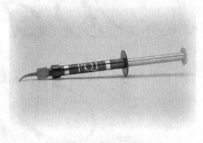 percent filled in an ethyl alcohol carrier. PQ1 is another great product that makes life in the treatment room easier for everyone. If you are concerned about cross-contamination of the syringes in the treatment room, Ultradent has a solution for that as well. Ultradent Syringe Covers are designed to cover the syringe during each use to prevent cross-contamination and to make your life easier in the sterilization area of the office. This is a nifty system that utilizes a small impulse sealer and has really made our sterilization system much simpler. So, give Ultradent a call at (800) 520-6635 to order PQ1 and the syringe covers. Do yourself a favor and get Ultradent's latest catalog today.

Pearl Forty-eight

OptiBond Solo
by Kerr

F or those who like the OptiBond technique, Kerr now has simplified things greatly. First off, you get filled technology for better adhesion and better microleakage protection—the same you expect from the OptiBond you have come to know. So, you don't risk any problems with bond strength. Secondly, you get a new, one-step system that saves you time (fewer steps) and money. That's great news, but I saved the best for last. Not only are there fewer steps to greater bond strength, but you get the slickest dispensing system you ever saw. It's a great, new, unidose system that looks like a rocket. You twist the head off the "rocket," and you have a container with one-tenth of a milliliter

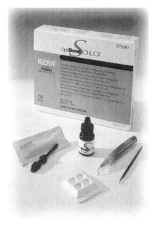

of OptiBond ready for dispensing with your Microbrush. There is no way that you can dispense one-tenth of a milliliter from a dropper bottle, so there is less waste with the unidose system. It comes packaged in a foil wrapper with the "rocket" inside. Infection control is much better—you use it once and throw the whole thing away. The unidose system costs the same as the dropper-bottle system, but I bet I can treat more teeth with the unidose than you can with the dropper bottle! Contact your dealer or call Kerr at (800) KERR-123.

Pearl Forty-nine

Prime & Bond NT
by Dentsply/Caulk

As most of you probably already know, Prime & Bond has been my bonding agent of choice for a number of years now. The material has worked well for me—a good dentin seal; no sensitivity; my fillings, crowns, and veneers don't come out; and it is easy to use (especially with the new bottle). Just when you think you have the perfect product, along comes an improvement that makes it even better. Caulk has done just that by adding a filler to Prime & Bond. You would expect that this adds to film thickness, but it does not, thanks to the magic of "Nanofillers." The NT means "Nanofiller Technology." Nanofillers are 100 times smaller than the fillers in hybrid composites. This gives you a stronger resin matrix, a

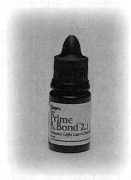

reinforced hybrid zone, and higher bond strength at the critical point where it is needed to withstand the stress of polymerization shrinkage of the restorative material. So much for all the technical stuff. What this means for everyday bonding is a material that, in my hands, offers the convenience of a true one-coat, one-cure application. Simply put, you get a better foundation. With one coat, I quickly and easily see the glossy surface that I am looking for. It seems to me that I have found a material that gives me a faster, easier, better way to place a bonding agent. Try Prime & Bond NT for yourself. I think you will like it, too. Order from your dealer or call Dentsply/Caulk at (800) 532-2855.

Pearl Fifty

OptiBond Solo Plus™
by Kerr

O ptiBond Solo Plus™ has added more filler to the bonding agent to better protect against microleakage. This added filler makes it faster and easier to apply the bonding agent to the tooth. This is a tricky material to describe. The filler seems to make the material thicker as you are applying it. You get that glossy look to the tooth very often with only one coat of the material. Here comes the tricky part. The resulting film thickness after you have light-cured the bonding agent is only 10 microns. So you 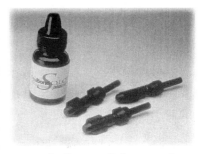 now can use OptiBond Solo Plus™ to seat indirects (inlays, onlays, veneers, crowns, and posts) without an additional activator or multiple coats. I like this system because it is so simple to use. Apply, lightly dry, light-cure, and you are finished. OptiBond Solo Plus™ is available in either the traditional bottle or in the nifty single-unit dose (the famous rocket). Order from your dealer or call Kerr at (800) KERR 123.

$\mathcal{P}earl$ $\mathcal{F}ifty\text{-}one$

Prompt®
by ESPE

I am not sure who keeps track of the generations of all the bonding agents, but this one is being referred to as a "sixth generation" bonding agent. I can tell you this much-Prompt® is different from anything you have used before. ESPE has managed to put into one package all of the components of adhesive dentistry-etch, prime, and bond-all in

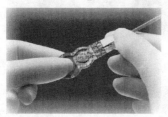

one neat little package with a built-in applicator. This is simply amazing. This is a unique chemistry system that makes bonding to dentin and enamel faster, easier, and better. Prompt® produces excellent, reliable bond strengths to dentin and cut enamel. With this system, there are no more worries about moist dentin or possible collagen collapse, because your etching, priming, and bonding are accomplished before drying. Rhonda, my clinical assistant, loves this product because of its simplicity! When a procedure calls for bonding, she simply picks up one or two packs of Prompt®. No more tubes of etch with tips, no more bonding wells, no more bottles of bond with caps to be removed, no more applicators, no more rinsing. Prompt® has eliminated all of this. Prompt® is a true single-step adhesive. The package for this remarkable bonding agent is called L-Pop®, because it resembles a lollipop. The package has three separate chambers. To activate, you simply compress the red chamber with your thumb and finger and force the liquid into the yellow chamber. While keeping pressure on the red chamber to prevent the material from back-flowing, you simply bend the red chamber onto the yellow chamber and compress the yellow into the green chamber. Prompt® now has been activated and is ready for use. Do not remove the applicator prior to activation. You now apply Prompt® to the tooth for 15 seconds using the microbrush applicator supplied, and then gently evaporate with air. It is not necessary to light-cure. You can begin placing your light-cured composite or compomer. One caution-read the instructions and follow them carefully. This material is not meant for use with dual-cured resins. There is one more giant advantage to using Prompt®! No more sensitivity! Yes, you heard me correctly-no more sensitivity. Prompt® will virtually eliminate the potential for post-operative sensitivity. This should be your bonding agent of choice. Order from your dealer or call ESPE at (800) 344-8235 or visit www.espeusa.com for more information.

Pearl Fifty-two

Dentastic Uno
by Pulpdent

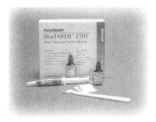

Here is a simple, quick, and easy material to use as a bonding agent. The good news is that it is less that half the price of other materials. The directions call for applying two coats of the material, but I have found that one application seems to produce a glossy surface on the dentin. I have not had any sensitivity with Dentastic Uno. Give it a try; I think you will like it. Order from your dealer or call Pulpdent Customer Service at (800) 343-4342 for more information.

● ●

Pearl Fifty-three

Seal & Protect™
by Dentsply/Caulk

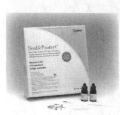

Hardly a day goes by that our office is not confronted with root-surface sensitivity. It will vary from the patient who complains of slight sensitivity to the one who must use warm water to rinse his mouth. I have tried every product that comes onto the market claiming to have solved the problem, but have had mixed feelings about them. Some require patient compliance to get the desired result, and that is always a mixed bag. The reason for this long introduction is to tell you about this new product from Caulk that is clinically proven to prevent dentinal hypersensitivity for up to six months. Seal & Protect™ is a light-cured dentin sealant designed to reduce thermal, chemical, and tactile hypersensitivity in exposed root-surface dentin. Seal & Protect™ will infiltrate and seal exposed dentin tubules, which reduces sensitivity and also reduces the continued wear of cervical dentin. The good news is that acid etching is NOT necessary, so in most cases you will not need to use an anesthetic. The procedure is to very carefully clean uninstrumented dentin with a rubber cup and nonfluoride cleaning paste. Rinse the area thoroughly, isolate well, and blot dry with a moist cotton pellet-this is to provide a "moist" dentinal surface. In other words, remove the excess moisture without desiccating the dentin. Open the bottle and dispense two or three drops into a clean well and promptly replace the cap. Then you simply apply Seal & Protect™ to the tooth, keeping it wet for 20 seconds. Then light-cure for 10 seconds, apply a second coat, and cure. Check for any excess on or below tissue and carefully remove. The patient will get instant relief that will last for up to SIX MONTHS. At the next hygiene appointment, one coat of Seal & Protect™ can be applied to renew the protection for another six months. This can be a great practice-builder because many patients don't know that sensitivity is treatable. In most states, Seal & Protect™ can be applied by a hygienist. The possibilities for this material are endless! How about sealing crown preps to reduce sensitivity with temps? Or how about sealing the margins of temporaries to prevent sensitivity? Those are just a couple of ideas that we thought of. Be sure to read and carefully follow instructions for best results. Order from your dealer or call Dentsply/Caulk at (800) LD-CAULK or visit www.caulk.com for more details.

Pearl Fifty-four

Gluma Desensitizer®
by Heraeus Kulzer

You all know about using Gluma® Desensitizer to stop sensitivity with a chairside procedure. If you are experiencing sensitivity with your composite restorations, then perhaps it is time to start using Gluma®. This simple, one-step procedure can be done in seconds, stopping the pain of localized sensitivity often associated with bonding procedures. It is easy to apply and is universally compatible with all materials. It will not interfere with the performance of resins, glass ionomers, or other

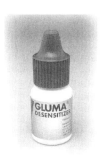

materials. Gluma® actually will increase the efficacy of whatever dentin bonding system you are using. Use it before you fill, seat crowns, inlays, veneers, or bridges. Order from your dealer or call Heraeus Kulzer at (800) 343-5336 for more information.

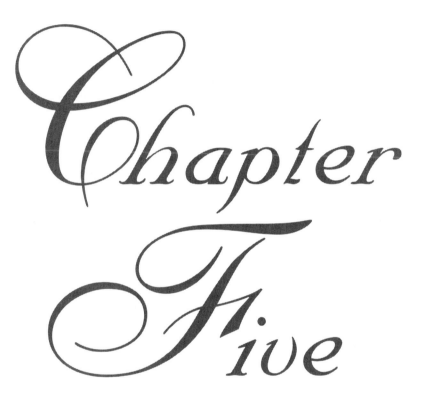

Chapter Five

Restorative, Cosmetic/Esthetic Dentistry

● ●

Pearl Fifty-five

The Smile Catalog
by Dr. William Dickerson

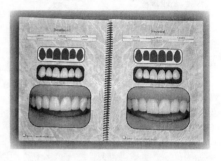

This is a great idea for communicating with the laboratory and for helping the patient determine the shape of his/her ideal smile. Other such smile guides used a lot of different models and, in my opinion, were too confusing for both the patient and the dentist. To simplify the selection of an ideal smile, Dr. Dickerson has used one patient and made 12 different sets of veneers to show how different combinations of anterior tooth shapes can be used to achieve the results. As you look through the Smile Catalog, the only thing that changes is the teeth; the lips and gingival tissues stay the same. The rather gender-neutral smile forces patients to choose the smile based on the shape of the teeth and not any other factor. Thanks for a great idea, Bill. If you are creating new smiles for patients in your practice, then you need the Smile Catalog. For additional information or to order, call Dr. Dickerson right away at (702) 878-1977.

Pearl Fifty-six

IPS Empress™
by Ivoclar Williams

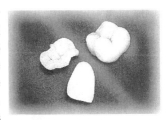

I have been using IPS Empress™ for over four years for veneers, inlays, onlays, and selected full crowns. I was first attracted to the technique by the wear characteristics of the material against natural dentition, and I have not been disappointed. The plus is exciting, new esthetic options with great-looking shades that make my finished product look really good. Empress has been a wonderful material to work with. Now, you can offer your patients the exceptional esthetic option of metal-free restorations. The all-ceramic Empress restorative system, with its unique leucite-reinforced ceramic material, offers exceptional esthetics and wear-compatibility (as I mentioned). You must follow the recommended preparation instructions to achieve exceptional marginal integrity. Those of you who have been impressed with other all-ceramic systems will marvel at the unparalleled beauty and natural vitality of Empress. The strength of the system is incredible. I have placed many of these restorations and have had only a handful of failures (that's less than five). In looking at the reasons for failure, most were due to the preparation of the tooth. I know that many of you already use this system, but I also know from the comments I receive around the country that many of you are reluctant to try nonmetal, reinforced crowns. I find that many of my patients complain of allergies to metals. The Empress material is biocompatible and will not cause allergy problems. So come on into the 21st century and try some of this wonderful material! You will not be disappointed with the results, and your patients will love the way their teeth look. Perhaps they will let you do even more Empress crowns in their mouths! For more information on IPS Empress™, contact your laboratory or call Ivoclar Williams at (800) 5-DENTAL.

Pearl Fifty-seven

Finesse All-Ceramic
From Dentsply/Ceramco

More and more dentists are looking for highly esthetic, metal-free restorations. Ceramco has introduced a new all-ceramic system that utilizes a pressable ceramic core system with innovative low-fusing porcelain. The system has significant clinical advantages, including strength, biocompatability, and marginal integrity. The

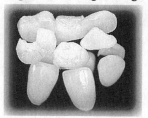

Finesse low-fusing porcelain gives you the advantages of superior wear characteristics, kindness to the opposing dentition, and chairside polishability. All of this on a beautiful, strong, pressed ceramic core. This is a system you should try. Check with your dental lab or call Dentsply/Ceramco at (800) 487-0100.

Pearl Fifty-eight

Symmetry Facial Plane Relator
by Clinician's Choice

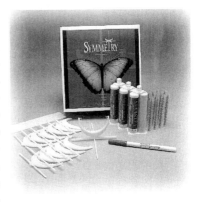

Peter Jordan has come up with another great product for the restorative practice to use in smile management. When planning an esthetic rehabilitation, it is essential that the midline of the new teeth coincides with the facial midline of the patient. Without something to guide the laboratory, this has often been difficult to achieve. With this new system, it becomes fast and easy! With the Symmetry Facial Plane Relator, the dentist can communicate an accurate measurement of the horizontal plane and the vertical plane for the dental laboratory. In just 60 seconds, the dentist can record an accurate bite registration, as well as the exact relationship of the patient's facial midline to his horizontal plane. All in one easy step. What a simple idea! For more information, call Clinician's Choice at (800) 265-3444.

Pearl Fifty-nine

Filtek P60 Posterior Restorative
by 3M ESPE

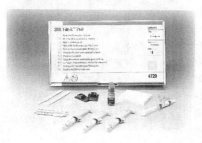

T his is 3M ESPE's entry into the packable posterior restorative field. This material has been extensively researched in the laboratory and in the field. I believe that 3M ESPE has combined some great posterior restorative handling characteristics. P60 packs well, and it resists slumping when you are carving before curing. It adapts well to margins and has a good flow and viscosity. The material does not stick to instruments, so you don't have to struggle with pull-back. P60 finishes well and does not require any special finishing materials to get a great shine. Much of what I have said could also be mentioned of some of the new posterior composites. The big news with P60 is that you can place it faster than any other material. You can place it in increments of 2.5 mm and cure it in just 20 seconds. Yes, that's right—half of the time required with other bulk-fill restoratives. Stop by the 3M ESPE booth and take a look at this material. P60 has all of the characteristics that I look for in a great posterior restorative. Order from your dealer or call 3M ESPE at (800) 634-2249 or visit their web site at www.3M.com/ESPE.

Pearl Sixty

Esthet-X™ Micro Matrix Restorative
by Dentsply/Caulk

Esthet-X™ falls into the category of the new "universal composite" systems. The "Micro Matrix" means that the particle size is smaller, to give the material a brilliant, durable polish that is comparable to the microfills. The material also has the physical properties of an advanced hybrid composite and thus can be used on posterior teeth. This material has combined the best of the hybrids and the best of the microfills into one great new product. Esthet-X™ is nonsticky for easy handling, and it is less sensitive to ambient light so you will experience a longer working time. The material is

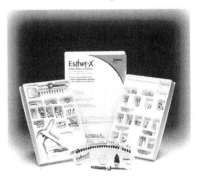

actually fun to work with because you can carve it and it resists slumping. It comes in 31 shades in three different opacities, so you can build very natural-looking teeth. Call Dentsply/Caulk at (800) 532-2855 or visit www.caulk.com. Order from your dealer.

Pearl Sixty-one

Point Four
by Kerr

Point Four is an optimized particle composite system of glass particles that are consistently in the range of .4 microns. By accomplishing this regularity in particle distribution and size, Kerr has produced a composite that has the strength of a hybrid and the polishability of a microfill. Now you can simplify your procedures by having just one product for all your composite needs. Point Four is a direct composite that can give you the esthetics through a wide variety of shades and a true chameleon effect for blending with adjacent teeth. I have used this material during a period of extensive field testing and have had excellent results in all areas of the mouth. If you are ready to reduce composite inventory, call your dealer and ask for Point Four. For more information, call (800) KERR-123 or visit their web site at www.kerrdental.com.

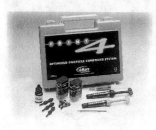

Pearl Sixty-two

Tetric Ceram
by Ivoclar Vivadent

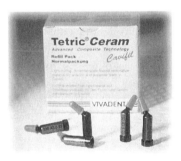

I came across this new material at the California Dental Association Meeting in Anaheim and have been using it since then. This is a new composite material that has outstanding handling characteristics. It allows you to do many of the things that you always have wanted to do with a composite, but were unable to do. Tetric Ceram demonstrates both stability of shape and ease of modeling. This means that you now can build a cusp or a marginal ridge or carve in some occlusal anatomy and expect the material to hold the form you have produced. You will have enough time to do this because the new catalyst system in Tetric Ceram prevents premature polymerization by operatory lights and ambient light. The material does not stick to your favorite composite instrument. The material has a continuous fluoride release similar to the compomers, and you will find that it is easy to finish to a very smooth surface and luster. Tetric Ceram has an outstanding radiopacity, which allows you to distinguish accurately between the restorative material and caries, and now you can see the smallest amounts of interproximal excess. The material is packaged in color-coded syringes and cartridges. Tetric Ceram definitely improves the everyday use of composites and makes it faster, better, and easier. Call Ivoclar Vivadent for additional information at (800) 533-6825 and order from your dealer.

● ●

Pearl Sixty-three

SureFil
by Dentsply/Caulk

I n the race to find an alternative to posterior two-surface amalgams, Caulk has entered with a new product called SureFil. I became familiar with this product in its development stage, and I have been impressed by its handling characteristics. Research has shown that

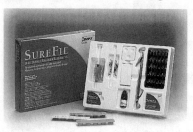

dentists have been looking for a nonamalgam restorative for Class II restorations that would allow them to easily achieve good contacts. Based on clinical trials and use in my office, I think SureFil deserves a serious look. The material handles like amalgam, thanks to a very precise assembly of different-sized glass particles. This "interlocking" action between the particles gives SureFil a feel and resistance similar to amalgam for ease of establishing contacts. You can actually pack the composite against the matrix band and see the band move. You also will find some other amazing differences with this product. It has an excellent depth-of-cure, which means that you can bulk-place the material up to almost 6 mm in depth. This means that most Class II restorations can be placed in bulk, carved, and cured in one step. You will need a curing light with an output of over 400 to achieve this, so be sure your curing light is operating at peak level. With the increased patient demand for esthetic restorations, it is great to have a new posterior composite with such good new characteristics. It is easy to handle, polishes well, and looks to me like it has great promise. Order SureFil from your dealer today.

● ●

Pearl Sixty-four

Prodigy Condensible
by Kerr Corporation

This is Kerr's entry into the "packable composite" market. Most of the packables now on the market have increased the particle size in order to achieve the resistance necessary to make it a packable. The current debate is whether these large particles cause shrinkage. In my practice, I have not detected any shrinkage of the packable materials.

Kerr has found a way to incorporate packability without increasing the size of the filler particles. Prodigy Condensible uses the same technology found in Prodigy and Herculite HRV hybrids. They have placed a unique additive in the resin that makes it packable. Since the particle size is not increased, Kerr is able to pack the material in a compule or unidose tip. This makes it much more convenient to dispense. A little more hand pressure on the dispensing gun is required, but it works well. It also is sculptable so that you can carve the material before curing it. Prodigy Condensible polishes nicely, and, with a good shade selection, it will give you a very esthetic result. You can order from your dealer or call Kerr Corporation at (800) KERR-123.

• •

Pearl Sixty-five

Revolution Flowable Light-Cure Composite
by Kerr Corporation

Since its introduction as the first flowable composite five years ago, Revolution has become the proven performer for versatile chairside convenience. Place your composite right where you want it and have it stay there without slumping or pulling back. Deliver the material via a 1 cc syringe with a disposable needle tip. It's amazingly simple! Use it for Class III and V restorations and for those teeth that you prepped with air abrasion. Finishing and polishing time and effort are cut radically because of the precise delivery created with the syringe. Revolution also can be used as a pit-and-fissure sealant, cement for veneers, and for many other applications. There is not a day in my practice that I don't ask my assistant to hand me the Revolution. The applications I find for this flowable resin increase with every use. Run, don't walk, to your dealer and order this material, or call Kerr Corporation at (800) KERR-123.

Pearl Sixty-six

Versaflo
by Centrix

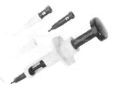

A re you tired of trying to disinfect your flowable composite syringe? Maybe you should look for a replacement. Versaflo is a practical solution to a light-cured flowable composite in a prefilled tip. Its versatility and ease of use can't be beat. Versaflo is the new single-dose, light-cured flowable composite that has a wide range of uses. It has a great viscosity that does not slump, and the material stays where you put it. Couple this with great shades and you have an unbeatable filling material for your conservative Class I preps, small Class III, and Class V restorations. Versaflo is compatible with all composite bonding agents, and it contains fluoride. The Centrix Single-Dose Needle Tubes make precise placement easy. Their disposability eliminates cross-contamination. Use Versaflo for luting porcelain veneers, filling bubbles in temporary crowns, pit-and-fissure sealing, and more. Call Centrix at (800) 235-5862.

● ●

Pearl Sixty-seven

Fuji II® LC
by GC America

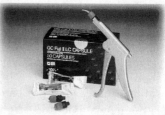

Fuji II® LC comes in premeasured capsules that are simple to activate and mix, giving you a consistent mix every time. It is a resin-reinforced glass ionomer restorative material that does not require a separate bonding agent. It will bond chemically to tooth structure in a wet field. It light cures in 20 seconds for immediate finishing. Fuji II® LC has a significant long-term fluoride release for protection against secondary caries. If you are looking for simplicity, esthetics, and economy, this is the product for you. If you are bonding glass ionomer to dentin before placing your composite restorations, this is an excellent choice. Order from your dealer or call GC America at (800) 323-7063 for more information.

Pearl Sixty-eight

Fuji IX™ GP
by GC America

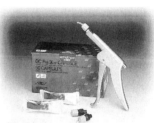

This product epitomizes what a pearl should be—faster, better, easier. Fuji IX™ is a packable glass ionomer restorative material. This material has to be the ultimate in restoratives for children. Since Fuji IX™ bonds directly to the tooth, you can use a simple, conservative restoration. There is no need for undercuts or fancy preps. Wonder of wonders, you do not need a bonding agent since this material is a glass ionomer and will bond to the tooth. Since this is a less invasive technique, you probably can get by with less anesthetic and, in some cases, no shots at all. Your kids will love that. The material is nonsticky, so you can quickly place it, pack it, and carve it. You have about two minutes of working time, and the material sets hard in about four-and-a-half minutes. So just place, pack, and finish—how easy can it be? Fuji IX™ is also a great choice for conservative air abrasion preps. Have you noticed that I haven't made any mention of curing lights? This material is self-setting, so you don't need one. The material is very wear-resistant and offers the superior fluoride protection of a glass ionomer. I also use the material as a temporary for emergency fillings and for core build-ups. Fuji IX™ comes in premeasured capsules, which I really like for the convenience and consistent mixes, or you can get it in a hand-mix power and liquid. Either way, if you are treating kids in your practice, you need Fuji IX™! Call your dealer or GC America at (800) 323-7063 or visit www.gcamerica.com.

● ● ● ● ● ● ● ● ● ● ● ● ● ● ● ● ● ● ● ●

Pearl Sixty-nine

Dyract
by Dentsply/Caulk

I am sure that everyone knows the primary advantages of glass ionomers are adhesion to tooth structure and fluoride release. Caulk now has introduced a product that combines these great glass ionomer properties with the advantages of a composite resin. In doing so, they have added a new word to your dental dictionary—"compomer."

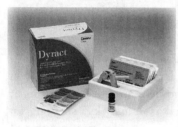

Caulk has established a new class of composite restorative, the compomer, a poly acid modified composite resin. The material first was introduced in Europe and has had a wide acceptance there for use in Class III and V restorations in adults and Class I and II restorations in children. The material is designed to work with Caulk's multipurpose bonding agent, Prime & Bond. In the development of Dyract, considerable emphasis was placed on the treatment technique. The result is a product that has excellent handling properties and time-saving benefits. While Caulk claims that you can skip the acid etch in Class V applications, I don't have that much confidence yet, and I still acid-etch before placing the Prime & Bond. The material is dispensed conveniently in a compule delivery system. Dyract's thick viscosity and lack of stickiness allows you to quickly place and easily contour the material in Class V cervical situations. In short, it is very easy to place. The shades are fantastic; the material blends so well with the tooth that it just seems to disappear. It is simple to finish, and the margins are excellent. You simply will not find a better product for Class V cervical restorations than Caulk's Dyract. One final note: Caulk still needs to find a better dispensing system for Prime & Bond! Order from your dealer or contact Dentsply/Caulk at (800) 532-2855.

Pearl Seventy

The Fissurotomy™ System
by SS White

Today's diagnostic methods do not always allow us to positively iden-
tify hidden caries. Sometimes, "watch and wait" was the most conservative decision. With the new SS White Fissurotomy™ System,
you don't have to watch and wait. The system includes a unique carbide
bur that can explore questionable pits and fissures. It is as simple to use as

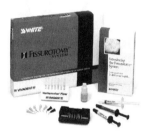

changing a bur in your handpiece, which is
actually what you do. The Fissurotomy™ tip
is extremely small (about the size of a 1/4
round bur), and it will quickly cut a minimally
invasive groove in suspicious fissures and pits.
Then you can make a definitive diagnosis and
treat the problem early on before it gets larger
and requires more involved treatment. No
need for new technology here; you use the skills that you already possess
with your high-speed handpiece. I found the system to be virtually pain-
free and very fast to restore, particularly when using my new electric high-
speed handpiece. I can have a quadrant of suspicious grooves and pits
done with ideal, conservative preps, filled and finished in about 10 minutes. More good news! Vivadent/ Ivoclar has partnered with SS White on
this kit, which includes Heliomolar® Flow. With exceptional flow properties and outstanding esthetics, Heliomolar® Flow is the ideal restorative
to use with the Fissurotomy™ system. Vivadent has maintained the
unique microfill chemistry of the original Heliomolar®, while making an
excellent flowable that will get into even the tightest spots. You can order
this all as a complete kit with the Fissurotomy™ burs and the Heliomo-
lar® Flow from your dealer or call SS White at (877) 779-2877 for more
information. An instructional video that clearly explains how the system
works is available with your purchase.

Pearl Seventy-one

Composi-Tight
by Garrison Dental Solutions, Inc.

T he biggest problem that composite-users have faced from the beginning is tight anatomical contacts. They have been hard to achieve. This is a great, new matrix system created just for composites that solves the problem of contacts. The system consists of small,

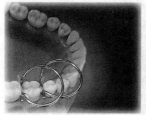

naturally contoured bands and a G-Ring that fits at the interproximal of the tooth. You place the band and wedge it. Then the G-Ring is placed into the interproximal area with rubber dam forceps. The force of the G-Ring will cause the contact to open slightly by pushing the two teeth away from one another. The result is an anatomically accurate contact at the tooth's natural height of contour. This is a real forward leap in the use of posterior composite materials. The G-Rings are unique in that they have burnished ends to grip the teeth at the gum line, thus keeping the bands and the G-Rings firmly in place. This ring will not spring loose and fly out of the mouth. With the Composi-Tight System, I am able to achieve a broad contact at the natural height of contour on the tooth. The G-Rings come in two lengths that allow you to do an MOD restoration or multiple restorations in the same quadrant. Dentists who seem to have thought of everything invented this system. If you are doing posterior, two-surface composites, you need the Composi-Tight System. To order, call (888) 437-0032.

Pearl Seventy-two

Matrix Systems for Composites
by Premier

This is not a single universal matrix, but a number of matrices to solve many of the problems associated with placing composite restorations. The first is the Stop-Strip, which is a Mylar-band strip that you can hold in place with one hand for Class III and IV restorations. Stop-Strips actually take you from three-handed dentistry to two. The secret is a unique plastic stop that is permanently attached to one end of the strip. You

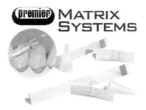

simply place the strip interproximally adjacent to the tooth you are filling and snug up the stop in the contact area. Now you can easily and quickly pull the strip tight against the composite with one hand while curing with the other. It also enables you to get your hands out of the way of the curing light so you have better access. Number two is the Strip-Aid, which is a self-adhesive proximal strip that will hold in place without using finger pressure. This allows you to cure without holding onto the strip. Number three is a favorite of mine, the Accor Matrix for core build-ups. This is a simple, cone-shaped matrix that can be quickly contoured with scissors to fit the gingival, and then easily cut to size for the required height. No lubrication is required; you simply cut the matrix away when the build-up is hard. You can use the Accor in the anterior or posterior with glass ionomers or composites. Number four is the nifty little Cure-Thru, which is a clear, cervical matrix for Class V restorations. The seven sizes are flexible enough to match the exact contour of the tooth and rigid enough to apply pressure needed for dense restorations with excellent marginal integrity. So there you have it:

matrix solutions to make composite placement faster, easier, and better! To place your order, call your dealer. For additional information, call Premier at (888) 773-6872 or visit their Web site at www.premusa.com.

Pearl Seventy-three

The Optilux 501
by Kerr/Demetron

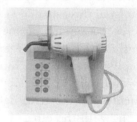

I have always been partial to curing lights by Demetron, because I am still using models that I bought in the early 1980s. The company recently has introduced the cure-all solution; a high-performance curing machine, which I feel is the value in quality light-curing. The 501 has a mode for virtually any curing you want to do: traditional curing in 10-, 20-, 30-, and 40-seconds, as well as continuous modes; ramp curing in a 20-second mode; bleaching in a 30-second mode; and a high-energy boost mode. This light will cure all composites and bonding agents on the market—guaranteed. The Optilux 501 offers a Boost 10-second cure mode, which will cure in excess of 4.7 mm deep. If you use the 8 mm turbo tip, you can cut that curing time in half. Dr. Ray Bertolotti refers to the Demetron turbo tip as the "poor man's laser." The 501 comes with a built-in digital radiometer that displays readings over 1,000mw/cm2, and a new filtering system prevents build-up of high heat generation. The 501 comes with the 8 mm turbo light guide and an accessory 11 mm light guide. It seems to me that the folks at Kerr/Demetron have thought of everything! To order, call your dealer. For additional information on the Optilux 501, call (800) KERR-123 or visit their Web site at www.kerrdental.com.

Pearl Seventy-four

Power Lite 100
by Spring Health Products

If you are looking for a new curing light with some great features, look no further; this is it! This curing light features a 12-volt, 100-watt lamp, which gives an extremely bright light. It's brighter than any other light on the market. There is a 10- to 90-second digital countdown timer, controlled and set by an on/off rocker switch, which is very handy. It will operate continuously for 15 minutes or more, allowing you to bond full-mouth brackets or upper and lower anterior veneers. Fan- 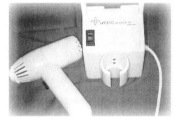 recycling will be a thing of the past. The curing light does not get so hot that it is uncomfortable to handle, as some lights do. It comes with mounting brackets and an autoclavable, 11 mm light guide. Also available are 13 mm straight, 8 mm curved, and 3 mm curved, autoclavable light guides. A radiometer is attached to the unit and is removable to test other lights. All of this costs much less than you would expect to pay. Ask your dealer or call Spring Health Products at (800) 800-1680. There is also a Highlight view light available.

Pearl Seventy-five

Curing Light 2500
by 3M

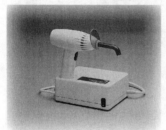

This new curing light is a hard-working, efficient light source that provides a reliable, affordable way to polymerize light-cured restorative materials. This light may not have all the bells and whistles, but it outperforms many lights in the same category. The 3M 2500 has a rotating nose cone that will rotate 360 degrees, making light-guide adjustment simple. This sounds so simple, but only this light has this handy feature. It makes putting the light guide exactly where you want it very fast and easy. It is amazing that no one has thought of doing this before. This model has a high-intensity light source that exceeds 800 mW/cm every time you turn it on. The ergonomically designed handpick easily stores in the base of the light unit. To keep you informed of the curing time, there is a 10-second audible beep. All in all, it's a very reliable light at an economical price. Order one today from your local dealer. You'll be glad you did.

Pearl Seventy-six

Light-Tip
by Denbur

I guess I am slow sometimes, but somehow this one got by me. What a great product! If it is used correctly, you can get tight contacts on your Class II composite restorations easily and consistently. The Light-Tip is a cone-shaped attachment that goes on the end of your curing-light wand, and the cone concentrates the light at the end of the tip. The cone is inserted from the occlusal into the resin in a typical Class II proximal box and then cured. This allows for curing of the most difficult area—the cervical margins. Composite does not

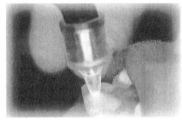

stick to the Light-Tips. I have found the tips to be very useful for tacking porcelain veneers, so that I can clear excess material and be certain the contacts are open before my final cure. Four sizes of Light-Tips are available to fit most curing-light wands. For more information, call Denbur at (800) 992-1399.

● ● ● ● ● ● ● ● ● ● ● ● ● ● ● ● ● ● ● ●

Pearl Seventy-seven

Esthetic Polishing System
by Brasseler

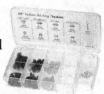

This is a "sandpaper disc" polishing system by Brasseler with some unique features. The disc attaches to the mandrel via a plastic material that does not allow the mandrel to come through the center of the disc. Now you have only polishing material in contact with the composite restoration. There is no metal center to nick or discolor the finish of the composite. The Brasseler system comes in two sizes and four grits. The coarse discs are safe-sided, and the other three sizes have grit on both sides of the disc. They cut well and have a good flexibility to allow you to get into those tight places. Another innovative product that makes our lives simpler! Call Brasseler at (800) 841-4522 to order or for details.

Pearl Seventy-eight

OneGloss and SuperBuff
by Shofu

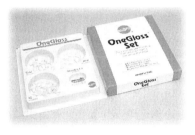

This is a new one-step composite polisher that is easy to use on all composites. This polisher finishes and then polishes simply by altering the contact pressure that you apply to the material. I find that OneGloss is unlike any other finisher and polisher on the market today. It is a very durable finisher and polisher and usually will last through the procedure. For convenience, it comes in three shapes (cup, inverted cone, and midi point) that quickly and easily snap onto a contra-angle mandrel. The OneGloss system is also less expensive than other systems currently on the market. So it qualifies under all four: faster, better, easier, and less expensive. Then combine the OneGloss with the new final polish for composites—SuperBuff—and you have the best of all worlds. SuperBuff is the first polisher on the market with a paste-impregnated disc. You do not have the mess of a syringe and the polish material splashing all over the place, including you and the patient. SuperBuff is easily activated by water or saliva, and it works with all composites on multiple surfaces. If you want a super polish, then get SuperBuff. Order from your dealer or call Shofu at (800) 82-SHOFU or visit their web site at www.shofu.com for more information.

Pearl Seventy-nine

Etch-Rite
by Pulpdent

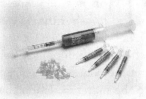

This is a 38 percent phosphoric acid etching gel for acid-etching dentin and enamel. So what, you ask— another etching material? The difference is in the packaging. Pulpdent has come up with a bulk package that we really like in our office. It comes with a 50 ml bulk storage syringe and five 3 ml empty syringes. The bulk syringe has a luer lock fitting that the 3 ml syringe locks into, so there is no possibility of leakage or any mess when refilling syringes. The kit includes 50 pre-bent tips for use with the 3 ml syringe. To order, call (800) 343-4342 or visit www.pulpdent.com.

Pearl Eighty

UltraEZ Desensitizing Gel
by Ultradent®

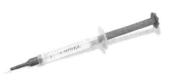

L eave it to the syringe people at Ultradent® to come up with great desensitizing gel in a very convenient dispenser that patients can use. UltraEZ is a 3 percent potassium nitrate and a 0.11 percent w/w fluoride ion- desensitizing gel that is designed for delivery in a custom tray. Use block-out resin to create reservoirs in the custom tray so that the gel is in contact with the sensitive area. This means quicker relief for your patients. The viscosity and stickiness of the gel allow the material to stay active for extended treatment times, if necessary, when it is used in a custom-fitted tray. Call Ultradent® at (800) 552-5512 to order.

Pearl Eighty-one

Pumice Preppies
by Whip Mix Corporation

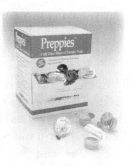

Finally! A simple, individual packet of PUMICE! Packaged just like your prophy pastes, this is unit-dose flour of pumice paste. It is ideal for use in cleaning the tooth surface prior to etching for restoration cementation. It is a cleaning agent that contains no flavoring agents, oils, or fluoride. Each cup provides enough flour of pumice paste for a single use, thus providing optimum infection control and savings by eliminating waste. Call and order from Whip Mix Corporation at (800) 626-5651.

Pearl Eighty-two

OsteoGraf/LD
by Dentsply CeraMed Dental

One thing that all extraction sites have in common is that there will be a loss of bone volume and dimension if the socket is not grafted. The restoring dentist should be responsible for ridge preservation and creating a good pontic site. This pure, porous, synthetic form of hydroxylapatite has been around for a while, but, unfortunately, suffers from a low level of awareness in the marketplace. It was previously known as Gen-Graft. It is probably one of the best-kept secrets in dentistry. When used as a bone-replacement material in extraction sites, OsteoGraf/LD has proven very effective in preventing alveolar ridge resorption and eliminating prosthetic problems associated with compromised esthetics of final restorations. This product has several unique qualities when compared to other similar products. First, it is the easiest product to use. OsteoGraf/LD is supplied in sterile 1- and 3-gram vials (I favor the 1-gram size), which can be reautoclaved up to three times. The vial interconnect accepts three different-style syringes that can be loaded easily with OsteoGraf/LD and then placed in the extraction site. You only use as much as you need, since the vial now can be sterilized and the remaining material used again. The material is extremely easy to handle and will stay where you put it after preparing the extraction site. The best news of all is that OsteoGraf/LD is very economical. The cost of the material is approximately $40 per gram, and an average of 1/3 to 1/2 gram is needed per extraction site. Compared to similar products on the market, OsteoGraf/LD is significantly more economical. Ridge resorption should be a thing of the past, because this should be your product of choice when grafting extraction sites. The technique is easily learned and will add only a couple of minutes to your extraction procedure. There is essentially no learning curve involved. Any dentist who can remove a tooth can easily place OsteoGraf/LD bone in the extraction site and 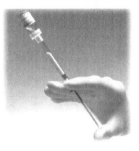 achieve the proper closure to maintain the patient's maximum ridge height. This is a great product that you should be using on every extraction every day! Call Dentsply CeraMed Dental at (800) 426-7836.

Pearl Eighty-three

PerioGlas
by Block Drug Corporation

Tooth removal causes unavoidable and unpredictable shrinkage of bone and soft tissue. As restorative dentists, we are more often than not confronted with a poor pontic site, which results in an unaesthetic replacement. I was referring out all my extractions, but now I am doing them myself. I made the decision that I was going to be in control of ridge preservation, because I know more about esthetic ridge design. I have come across another great product to get the results you want. PerioGlas is an osteo-productive ceramic material used for bone regeneration. The material is fast and easy to use. The material comes in a sealed container and takes only seconds to prepare. It contains a broad particle-size range of 90 to 710 microns to opti-

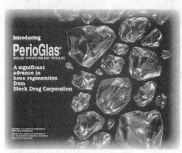

mize compactibility. The material will bond to both bone and soft tissue. PerioGlas is easy to mix, and the material will not slip off instruments when you are picking it up or transporting it to the mouth. It is easy to pack with an instrument. Since it is hemostatic, as you pack the material, the bleeding in the extraction site stops. This prevents the material from being dislodged by subsequent bleeding. You can use a cotton roll to blot the material and further pack the site. The material will not float out of the defect site. It is unaffected by adjacent suctioning. PerioGlas definitely is a material that you will want to try if you are concerned about ridge preservation. I have found it to be fast to use with predictable results. Order from your Block Drug Dental Consultant or call (800) OK-BLOCK.

Pearl Eighty-four

IntegraPost System
by Dental Logics

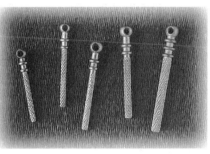

This is a titanium alloy post that gives you biocompatibility and strength. It has a surface with hundreds of raised facets that allow the cement to integrate with the post to form a powerful interlocking bond within the canal. The head of the post is uniquely designed with three holes that make it one of the easiest posts to handle. You simply use the IP Carrier to engage the cross hole and carry the post to the tooth. The flow-through head of the post also allows build-up material to integrate with the post head. Call (800) 778-0075 for details.

$\mathscr{P}earl\ \mathscr{E}ighty\text{-}five$

Luscent Anchor ™
by Dentatus USA

A nonmetallic fiberglass-resin post, Luscent Anchors are particularly for anterior cases where you want to restore the tooth with a non-metallic crown and avoid the possibility of metal compromising your shade. This is an extremely simple system from Dentatus. It is available in three diameters to fit small canals and large canals.

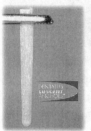

I often have a concern about polymerization of the resin material I am cementing my post with. Did the light reach into the canal? The Luscent Anchors™ will transmit polymerizing light into the canals, so I am sure that the material has cured. They are compatible with all restorative materials. You can do a post and core very quickly. The anchors reflect the colors of your restorative materials. You can choose whatever shade you want for your final crown or veneer. Research is showing that this type of post is much less likely to cause a root to crack. Call Dentatus USA at (800) 323-3136 to place your order.

Pearl Eighty-six

Optipost System
by Brasseler

I know what you are thinking: this is just what we need—a new post system. Don't we have enough already! Well, this one is special. The Optipost System is a tooth-specific restorative system that is color-coded to make its use very simple. The titanium Optiposts are individually sized to fit coronally destroyed anteriors, cuspids, and bicuspids on the upper and lower. They all have the advantages of a cast post at a fraction of the cost. The preparation system has been simplified greatly to make the placement of this system fast and easy. Due to the pyramid design of the post and the close adaptation to the root canal wall, it is well-retained. In the design phase, the ideal tooth anatomy was studied carefully to provide the correct post shape for each tooth. This design offers an optimal distribution of forces, giving maximum resistance to fracture. It is a system you should try. Call Brasseler at (800) 841-4522.

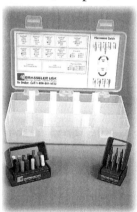

$\mathcal{P}$earl $\mathcal{E}$ighty-seven

Nifty Strip
by HIT, Inc.

T his mylar matrix strip is THE solution to getting great adaptation for anterior restorative materials. This has got to be one of the most significant advances in anterior restorations in a long time. How many times have you struggled trying to get mylar matrix

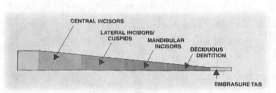

strips to fit both the gingival and the incisal part of the anterior tooth you are trying to restore? I know I have had a lot of problems with them. It always seems like you have to compromise something. Now comes the solution—Nifty Strip (what a great name)! The patented taper allows the Nifty Strip to coincide exactly with the vertical dimension of any tooth. It conforms to the tooth surface with no kinks in the foldover, thus eliminating excessive trimming and giving us a better restoration. It has great stability, too. When incisal placement is difficult, place the Nifty Strip through the embrasure using a floss threader. I keep finding more uses for it as we use it. This is definitely a terrific find. Call HIT, Inc. at (800) 472-5409 to order.

Pearl Eighty-eight

Accu-Prep™ Deluxe
by Bisco

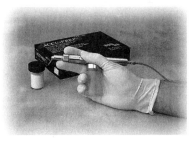

I know what you are thinking: "I already have a sandblaster." But this one is different! Accu-Prep™ operates at only 40 p.s.i. and features a springless, air-activated on/off button for ease of cleaning. It is constructed of stainless steel, so it keeps looking great. Accu-Prep™ is designed to mechanically enhance bond strength to porcelain, cast alloys, amalgams, and composites. If you are doing any cosmetic dentistry, you need one of these. The nozzle rotates 360° for access to intra- and extraoral surfaces. Here's the best part...Bisco has made Accu-Prep™ with a quick-disconnect that allows the entire unit to be autoclaved. Call Bisco at (800) BIS-DENT for more info.

Pearl Eighty-nine

Snoop Caries Detecting Dye
by Pulpdent

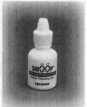

One of the problems I have had with caries-detecting dyes is that all of them are red. The red color of these dyes makes it difficult to see what you want to see. Someone must have been listening. Pulpdent has introduced a dye that is blue (what an innovation!) and is easy to read, due to the excellent color contrast to the tissue we work with. As with most materials we use, Snoop is not perfect and must be used with care, because the dye can stain the tissue. I find that if I use a Microbrush, I can apply the Snoop just where I want it and not have any problems. This is a simple, quick, and easy product to use. Thanks for listening, Pulpdent! Order from your dealer or call Pulpdent at (800) 343-4342.

Pearl Ninety

MicroDose
by Premier Dental Products

I am becoming more interested in single-use packaging from an infection-control point of view and to simplify the treatment area. The folks at Premier have taken a number of the everyday products we need for adhesive dentistry and packaged them as "Single Patient Applicators." What a great idea! The applicators are easy-to-use plastic containers with a convenient small tip to place the material where you want it. I use the following applicators: Therma-Trol, which is a desensitizer gel; Porcelain Etchant, which is a 9.6 percent hydrofluoric; Porcelain Silane, which gives you a fresh silane that has not been contaminated by exposure to air; and Chlorhexi Prep, which is a full 2 percent chlorhexidine liquid that is a great preparation disinfectant. I am sure that more of the products we use on an everyday basis will become available in single-use packaging. Order from your dealer; call Premier Dental Products at (888) 773-6872 for details or visit www.premusa.com.

Chapter Six

Crown and Bridge Restorative

Pearl Ninety-one

The Block Inlay Bridge
by Aesthetic Porcelain Studios

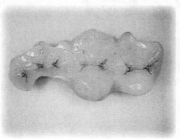

We all have been searching for the conservative, esthetic inlay bridge for years. I had limited success with the Maryland bridge, and the esthetics certainly left something to be desired. Today, patients are becoming more and more demanding. They question why we must prepare teeth for full coverage, and they expect the same vitality, chroma, and hues that they have in their veneers or all-ceramic crowns in their crown and bridge restorations. They also question the appearance of metal margins on porcelain-fused-to-metal cases. The Block inlay bridge solves these problems. The inlay bridge has a metal substructure that is embedded in the porcelain (or composites) for strength. Your preparations are the same as a gold inlay bridge, but with no undercuts, and they must be parallel. I have seated a number of these bridges, and they are fantastic. David Block has come up with a winner. I have even used the bridge in the anterior and have achieved optimal esthetics with the proper preparation of the teeth. To date, David has fabricated more than 1,000 of these bridges with a zero-breakage factor. The next time you are looking for an alternative, call David at Aesthetic Porcelain Studios at (800) 544-9605.

Pearl Ninety-two

The C-LECT Crown
by Keller Dental Laboratories

This is a great crown that I have been using in my practice for about four years. I have placed close to a thousand of these crowns, and they are absolutely beautiful! The C-LECT crowns fit extremely well, because the three processes that can cause the most errors have been eliminated in the creation of this product. There is no waxing, no investing, and no casting to cause distortion in the metal coping. The precision-fit copings of 24k gold are formed directly on your die by an electroplating process. The marginal accuracy and coping retention are superior to cast metals. That's all good news, but here comes the 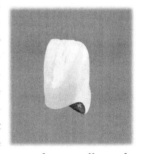 best feature of these crowns: The esthetics are re-created naturally and beautifully in the C-LECT crowns. The vital dentin hues are created without opacity because of the warm yellow color of the gold coping, so the shades are simply breathtaking. So now you have it…the perfect combination of fit, strength, and great shades. I almost forgot—since oxides will not form on the 24k gold, you will not see gray shadow or dark margins at the gingival. When I first started prescribing these crowns, I always asked for porcelain butt margins. Now, I do not feel they are necessary. Keller gives a seven-year, no-breakage guarantee with these crowns. How can you lose? Call Keller Dental Laboratories at (800) 325-3056 for additional information or to receive mailers.

Pearl Ninety-three

Procera
by Nobel Biocare USA

I have had the opportunity to use the Procera AllCeram crowns. Unlike other all-ceramic crowns, this one has been developed with extra strength for every position in the mouth, even in the posterior. This means you can eliminate the PFM crown in the posterior and get rid of metal allergies. Those ugly dark or discolored margins will be

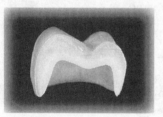

a thing of the past with this unique crown. The process of making this crown has eliminated three of the areas that cause laboratories the most problems in controlling the quality of their products, namely, waxing, investing, and casting. The coping is computer-machined directly onto the die. You can use conventional preparation techniques, and only a 1 mm chamfer prep is required. There are no cementation restrictions, so you can use your favorite cement. The shades are fantastic. In areas where you need more strength, this is a great choice. One drawback: You must allow some extra lab time for the process. Call Procera at (800) 891-9191 for the address of a lab that belongs to the Procera Network.

$\mathscr{P}earl$ $\mathscr{N}inety\text{-}four$

IPS Empress2
by Ivoclar North America

voclar has just introduced a new Empress material for three-unit bridges that has improved upon the great characteristics of IPS Empress. With additional strength and increased fracture toughness, IPS Empress2 is indicated for anterior all-ceramic bridges and full-coverage anterior and posterior single units.

The new material is for full-coverage three-unit bridges from the second bicuspid forward with a single pontic. This new-found strength results from a change in the formulation of the chemical structure. The Ivoclar chemists can explain this much better than I can. This new glass ceramic material allows for some great shading, so it is about as close to natural tooth color as you can 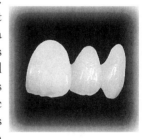 get. You now can create more biocompatible restorations, and your ceramist can achieve more natural results. Research has shown the IPS Empress2 material to exhibit the lowest wear of antagonist tooth structure of any ceramic on the market today. Your IPS Empress lab will be able to use a similar "press" technology and the same equipment as the IPS Empress system. IPS Empress2 can be adhesively bonded to the tooth or, in situations that do not permit an adhesive bond, you can cement with ProTecCEM, a new low-expansion hybrid-ionomer cement or a glass-ionomer cement. A great combination of strength, great natural-looking shades, adhesive bonding, and low-wear characteristics makes this an exciting new product for the "esthetic revolution!" Order from your lab, or call Ivoclar North America at (800) 533-6825 for more info. Do it now!

$\mathcal{P}$earl $\mathcal{N}$inety-five

The Dental Button
by Advantage Dental Products

I absolutely could not practice dentistry without this incredible, little crown matrix button. The button is a small, round piece of thermoplastic that softens when heated. I soften the button in hot water from the instant hot-water faucet that I installed in my operatory (like 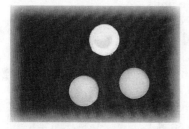 the one for coffee in hotel rooms). Then you form the soft material around the tooth or teeth to be prepped and extend to teeth on either side for stops. Blow air to harden and remove. Presto! In less than 30 seconds, you have a perfect, hard-plastic mold, with incredible detail, for making temporary crowns and bridges. The plastic still has some flexibility, which makes it easy to handle. It is more accurate, easier, and less expensive than alginate, putty, wax, or anything else you use to fabricate a matrix. Make a custom-made temporary in a fraction of the time it takes you now. Call Advantage Dental Products at (800) 388-6319 and order some today!

Pearl Ninety-six

Luxatemp Automix Plus System
by Zenith

You should be aware by now that a big change is occurring in cartridge systems that we use to mix and deliver materials in dentistry. All cartridge systems and dispensing guns are changing. The new cartridges will not be compatible with the old dispensing guns. It will no

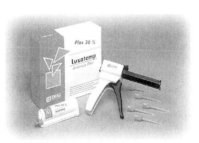

longer simply be a matter of changing the slide in order to accommodate a new temporary material or a new impression material. Out with the old guns; in with the new. That's the bad news! The good news is that the new cartridges are stronger and usually larger. That is what has happened to my favorite bis-acryl temporary material—Luxatemp. The Automix Plus cartridge holds 30 percent more material, and the small catalyst port that has caused many of you problems in the past has been eliminated. The dispensing ports have been made larger and have been separated to eliminate cross-contamination of materials and clogging of the ports. This is an extremely important change in this delivery system because all of the waste has been eliminated. It no longer is necessary to bleed the cartridges each time before placing a new tip. This eliminates the most common excuse not to use a bis-acryl temporary material. Now, when you open a new Luxatemp cartridge, you bleed the cartridge once and place a tip. Deliver the mixed material into your matrix and make your temporary. Now you can remove the tip and replace the cap. The next time the cartridge is used, it is not necessary to bleed the material when you remove the cap and put on a new tip. Wow! What a great improvement. The new Luxatemp Plus cartridge fits quickly and easily into the new dispensing gun that was designed

● ●

with the clinical assistant in mind. The new dispensing gun has a material flow with much less trigger pressure required. The new tips are smaller and more compact, which results in less air being incorporated into the temporary. This means you will have fewer bubbles and voids in your temporaries. Well done, Zenith. You have taken a superior temporary material and made it even better. Now you can eliminate the messy, smelly methyl methacrylates from your office and make the change to the best temporary material on the market. Take advantage of the introductory specials and order today from your dealer. Call Zenith at (800) 662-6383 for more information.

Pearl Ninety-seven

E-Z Temp Inlay and E-Z Temp Onlay
by Cosmedent

I want a temporary that is consistently easy to handle, quick to place, easy to get the bite right, a decent shade, doesn't require cementing, little or no sensitivity for the patient, does not come out between appointments (but is easy to remove at the seating appointment), and one that can be placed by either the dentist or an auxiliary. This

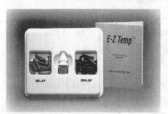

inlay/onlay kit from Cosmedent does all of the above. E-Z Temp is a light-cured temporary restorative designed for inlays and smaller, one-cusp onlays. The material is quick and easy to place—you don't even need a matrix. As you light-cure the material, it will expand enough to seal the cavity, protect the tooth, and prevent sensitivity. After the material is set, you can actually carve it (it will feel like you are carving soap). It has excellent retention, but is quick and easy to remove and leaves no residual in the tooth, so the cavity is clean and ready for try-in or etch. This is one of those materials that you can sit around and think of many more uses for. For instance, use it to close endo access (all endodontists should have some E-Z Temp in their offices and get rid of that awful stuff they use that is so hard to remove); use it to seal implant screw access between appointments; use it for emergency lost fillings; the list is endless. The E-Z Temp onlay material is a stiffer version for better retention with larger restorations. You can order E-Z Temp in a unit dose kit or in syringes. I couldn't practice without this one! Order your kit from Cosmedent by calling (800) 621-6729.

Pearl Nighty-eight

Flexible Clearance Tabs
by Belle de St. Claire

Many times, it is very difficult to check the amount of occlusal clearance when prepping posterior teeth for crowns or inlays. These Flexible Clearance Tabs make checking that clearance very easy and consistent. The "Flex Tabs" come packaged in three 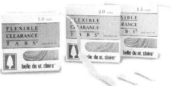 thicknesses—1.0mm, 1.5mm, and 2.0mm—with 25 disposable tabs in a dispenser box. Just place in the mouth over the prep, have the patient bite, and pull on the tab. If it pulls through, you know the clearance is OK. No more guessing—use this quick and easy way! For additional information or to place your order for "Flex Tabs," contact your dealer.

Pearl Ninety-nine

EZ Contact
by APS Block Dental Technologies

O ne of the most frustrating things for me in doing crowns and bridges is contacts. Both loose and tight contacts are a problem. If the contact is loose, I must send it back to the lab to add porcelain to the contact and reappoint the patient. How do I communicate to the lab how much to add? Very difficult! If the contact is tight,

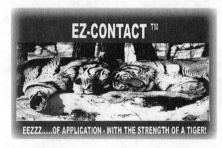

then everyone holds their collective breath while I slowly and carefully adjust the contact, only to find that I have taken too much and it must go back to the lab. My friend, David Block at Aesthetic Porcelain Studios, has come up with a solution. He has developed a kit that you can use to bond a special composite to the porcelain to correct loose contacts. The kit includes porcelain etch, primer, bond, composite, and polishing materials. You also can use this material to add to pontics that no longer fit the tissue. I am sure that this will be one of those materials that I will find many uses for as time goes on. I think it is a great product that deserves your attention. I can save the patient another appointment by using this material. Call David at (800) 544-9605 to order.

Pearl One-hundred

VisionFlex
by Brasseler

I hope that by now you have tried the new VisionFlex discs. These are by far the best diamond discs to come on the market. You actually can see through the disc while it is turning, so you can now see what you are cutting with a disc. When my Brasseler rep, Charley Rose, told me this story, I thought to myself, "Yeah, sure, Charley, you must be exaggerating now!" But he was right; they are wonderful for shaping ceramics, acrylics, and stone. You must match the proper disc with each material. The discs allow optimum visibility and a great flexibility because they are so thin. They produce smooth surfaces that are polished easily with the Dialite system. Now, they have come out with a smaller-diameter disc that can be used in the mouth. This is particularly useful to make those small changes in porcelain or Empress crowns and veneers. Another great product from a great, innovative company! Call Brasseler today at (800) 841-4522 to order or for more information.

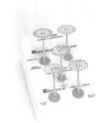

● ●

Pearl 101

Brasseler Polishing Products
by Brasseler

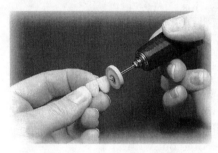

Dialite, the tremendous porcelain polishing system, has been expanded to include many other shapes. When the system first came on the market, the only shape available was a large-diameter wheel in the pre-polisher and the finisher. Brasseler has added a number of shapes to the line, until now there is a complete family of shapes and sizes. This is the only product that I am aware of that will easily restore a natural, high shine to porcelain without having to reglaze. Now, all of your porcelain-polishing needs are met using one of these instruments. The white prepolishers are available in all shapes as well. Brasseler also has a composite polishing system called Diacomp This is a two-step system that comes in three shapes — a point, a wheel, and a cup. The secret is a unique, diamond-impregnated surface that comes in medium and super-fine grits. The system is not meant for gross reduction, but I have found that you can put on a great finish very quickly. The system eliminates the need for extra instruments and pastes to put on the final high polish that is so necessary with composites. Try the Diacomp system. I think it will surpass your expectations. To order, call Brasseler at (800) 841-4522.

$\mathscr{P}earl\ 102$

The Great White Gold Series Burs
by SS White

W ow! What a cutting devil this bur is! About six years ago, SS White came out with its restoration-removal burs, which were great. Apparently, a lot of us started using them for other procedures and began wanting some other shapes and designs. This company listens! The result is an expanded Gold Series set of burs. These burs make it easy and quick to cut a hole in a crown for endo access. I had a problem with the original burs breaking at the neck when I tried to use them to remove crowns. Now, SS White has strengthened the neck and done 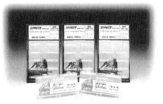 something to make the burs cut faster, because you can cut slots for crown removal really fast now. This is important if you are using some of the new cements that crown removers no longer work on. So, if you are looking for a bur that will make your procedures faster, get the new Gold Series burs from SS White today. Your satisfaction is 100 percent guaranteed, so how can you lose? Contact your SS White dealer.

$\mathcal{P}earl\ 103$

Autoclavable Aluminum Bur Blocks
by Brasseler USA

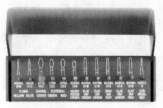

My clinical team tends to dislike the bur and diamond systems that I get from Brasseler, because they have a hard time remembering what diamonds and burs should be returned to which bur blocks after a procedure. They either have to ask me (I am usually no help), or they have to look in the catalog to compare the number with the shape. This really slows up the sterilization procedure and makes the team like the idea of disposable diamonds. Well, Brasseler is always trying to help dentists and their clinical teams by providing better products. Brasseler uses lasers to etch their bur blocks. It is an amazing process to watch at their factory in Savannah, Ga. Since they were already laser-etching the numbers on the blocks, the solution was to begin to etch the shape of the burs and diamonds on the blocks. Now all the team has to do is match up the shapes, and the burs and diamonds are quickly returned to their proper places. All new kits have this new etching. In a few months, you will be able to get customized laser-etched bur blocks for your own special selection of burs and diamonds. You can choose from a great variety of sizes and number of slots. Thanks, Brasseler, for another great solution! To order, see your local representative or call Brasseler at (800) 841-4522.

$\mathcal{P}earl$ 104

Shorter-Than-Short and New Finishing Strips
by Brasseler

Shorter-Than-Short is a system of diamonds that have a shank that is shorter than the standard short-shank burs. Many times, I have wished for a little less shank on a bur with a young child or an adult with severely limited opening. In fact, there were even times when I would cut off the shank with a "joe dandy" disc, but that did not work very well. Now, Brasseler has solved that problem with these new diamonds that are designed to be used in our small-head handpieces and come in a number of standard shapes and grits. Everyone should have one of these sets on the shelf. You never know when you will need it, and

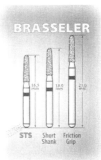

you certainly will be thankful when that unusual case comes in. So order a kit now. The other showstopper is a new Diamond Finishing Strip that is cleverly designed with holes in it. I assume that the idea came from the highly successful Vision Flex, the see-through diamond discs. The strips are very thin and the holes make them self-cleaning. With regular diamond finishing strips, debris tends to build up and clog the diamonds, making them less efficient. The strip also gets thicker and harder to handle. This problem is solved with this new strip. It is quick-cutting and easy to work with in a tight contact area, which is where I generally have a lot of problems. The holes also allow better vision of the filling or tooth you are shaping with the strip. This has already made a number of procedures easier and quicker. You need to call Brasseler at (800) 841-4522 and order some right away!

$\mathcal{P}earl\ 105$

Snap-Stone
by Whip Mix Corporation

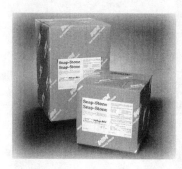

W hen you need a quick stone model, this should be your material of choice. We have been using it for about eight months now, and it is great. What makes it unique is a high, early compressive strength. You get an accurate working model in only five minutes. The problem with most quick-set gypsum products is that the teeth break off the model when you separate it. Not so with Snap-Stone! Use it for making custom trays for bleaching, mouthguards, vacuum-formed splints, temporaries, denture repairs, orthodontic appliances, and even study casts. Whip Mix Corporation will send you a free sample. Just call (800) 626-5651. One caution: Don't fool around when you mix it. Get your model poured quickly. It does set fast and hard. Order from your dealer.

$\mathcal{P}earl$ 106

Bite-Tab®
by Panadent Corporation

S omeone has finally invented a replacement for messy wax and compound materials for the bite fork on a face bow registration. Bite-Tabs® are self-adhesive compound discs to be applied to the bite fork when you are ready for a bite transfer. They are quick and easy to apply, and they remove just as easily with no messy cleanup. You may have to boil your present bite forks to be sure that they are very clean and that no wax build-up exists. The adhesive material in the Bite-Tab® will 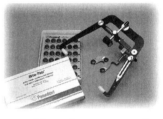 not stick to wax. They are universal and disposable. This is a simple, but really great idea for dentistry that certainly makes our job a lot easier and quicker. To order or for more information, call Panadent Corporation at (800) 368-9777 and ask for part number 4405.

$\mathcal{P}earl$ 107

The Crown Grabber II
by Kalmed Dental Products

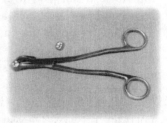

We always removed our temporaries with the Backhaus towel clamp. However, with the advent of stronger temporary materials, the towel clamp would no longer "grab" the crown. Len Jacobs recognized this and designed the Crown Grabber II, very descriptively named, because that is exactly what it does. And it does it extremely well! I have been using this instrument for over six months now, and it is great. It firmly grasps the temporary crown, and I simply wiggle the instrument slightly to break the cement bond, and out it comes easily and in one piece. We have found a number of other uses for the instrument, including placing permanent crowns for try-in and cementation, removing uncemented try-ins, and have even removed a couple of primary molars with it. This one is a no-brainer; you need to have a Crown Grabber II in your instrument set-up. So call Kalmed Dental Products at (800) 322-8815 and order one, or better yet, order three so you are never caught without one of these great instruments.

$\mathcal{P}earl$ 108

Crown-A-Matic
by Peerless International

O ne of the most perplexing problems is crown removal, but not with this crown and bridge remover! This instrument is extraordinarily simple to use and requires no assistance. How many times have you broken a tooth or the crown trying to remove it? Not with this one. Most crowns are removed with no damage to the tooth or the crown. The cement bond is severed by means of a short, but intensive, shock pulse. In most cases, the procedure is painless and is not frightening or

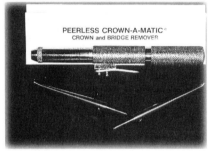

uncomfortable for the patient. I have been using this instrument for over 10 years now, and I can't tell you how many times it has saved me in a difficult situation. The instrument has been in constant use all that time and has never required any repair or maintenance. This is one that every dentist should have on the shelf. Don't wait. Get one today! Call Peerless International at (800) 527-2025.

$\mathcal{P}earl$ *109*

KY Crown Removal Pliers
by GC America

I was visiting with the GC America folks at the Chicago Midwinter meeting in February. They showed me many great, new products, but one was a product that they have had for a number of years. This is a nifty instrument for handling both temporary crowns and full

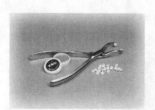 crowns. Since the bisacryl temporary crowns are very hard, it is difficult to remove them with the towel clamps that I once used. The sharp points just skip off the temps. The KY Pliers give a great grip and make temporary crown removal easy. For handling crowns, place rubber-packing material on the tips of the pliers to protect the crown. Next, dip the rubber tips into some emery powder that is supplied. This emery powder is like magic; the tips will not slip off the crown. I have found the pliers to be very effective for carrying crowns to the mouth for try-in and cementation and for removing crowns after trying them in. No more dropping crowns in the mouth because your gloves are slippery. No more struggling to get crowns off after you have tried them in the mouth...thanks to a wonderful instrument! Order from your dealer.

Pearl 110

The Easy Pneumatic Crown and Bridge Remover
by Dentco Research & Development Corporation

This crown and bridge remover actually is a handpiece that connects directly to your 2/3-hole- or 4-hole-style connector. The remover comes with three hooks to cover all situations and is activated by a button on the side of the handpiece. The remover's gentle, pneumatic operation is swift and subtle, so the cement bond gets the impact, not the patient. You can use a fine-tuning adjustment to give you complete control. Patients seem to tolerate the procedure very well and quite often do not know that the crown or bridge is out. I have found that it works well on bridges and on 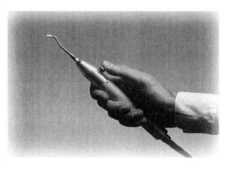 crowns if you can get hold of a margin. The remover is completely autoclavable and comes with a 30-day trial. Call Dentco Research & Development Corporation at (800) 454-9244.

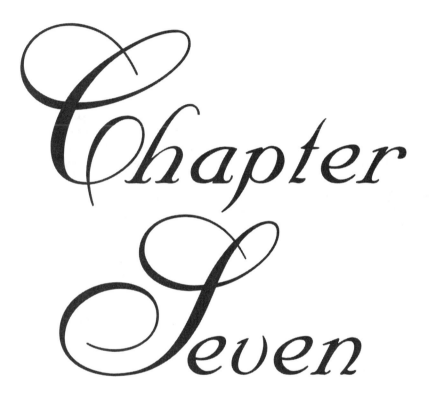

Chapter Seven

Impressions

$\mathcal{P}earl$ *111*

Imprint II
by 3M ESPE

W hat? Another impression material? Yes, but read on. 3M ESPE has a winner with this one. I have been using Imprint II on a daily basis since it was introduced at the CDA meeting in Anaheim. This material is one of the new, two-phase systems utilizing a

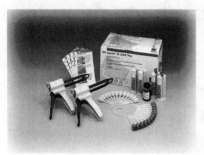

wash material and a tray material. As you know, if you follow "Pearls," I use Kerr Extrude as my benchmark impression material. 3M ESPE has made a number of changes in its material-dispensing systems. The tray material has a very high viscosity and is very heavy-bodied, but it has excellent elastic recovery, high tear strength, and dimensional stability. To save our dental assistants' hands and forearms, 3M ESPE has developed a new dispenser that has 40 percent more extrusion power. That means you need less hand force to operate the dispenser. My dental assistants love it because it is so easy to use! There are two wash materials to choose from—a low viscosity or a regular viscosity. In my hands, I tend to favor the regular viscosity material. The wash material is meant to be dispensed from the "gun," which required a technique change for me. I have adapted to using 3M's tips on the dispenser and found that it saves time and gives me more control in placing the material. Neither the low nor the regular viscosity washes slump or drip off the tooth. Imprint II sets in the mouth in four minutes, which saves time and is more comfortable for patients. The cartridges are labeled showing working and oral set times, and they are color-coded for easy matchup with the color-coded tips. The cartridges have dual ports that keep the two materials separate and virtually eliminate plugging. You can reap the cartridge and throw away the tip immediately after use, preventing cross-contamination and promoting infection control. I have had great success with my impressions—the model work looks very good and the resulting crowns, bridges, and inlays fit well. Now is a good time to try this product since 3M is offering incentives. Call 3M's tech hotline at (800) 634-2249 for more information or order from your dealer.

Pearl 112

Take 1
by Kerr

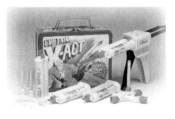

Kerr's hydrophilic vinyl impression material is being marketed in a creative way—an action character named Captain X-Act. Take 1 is a serious entry into the impression-material field with a new hydrophilic formula that will make great impressions even in the wettest of fields and a fantastic impression in a dry field. It comes in a nice variety of washes and tray materials to suit every technique. A free-flowing wash material comes in a fast and regular set that can be combined with a regular- or fast-set tray material or a rigid fast-set tray material. I favor the medium monophase fast-set material with the fast-set tray material. In my hands, I got the best results with this combination. Take 1 resulted in excellent impressions in areas that I would consider compromised by blood and saliva. I normally would not take an impression in a contaminated field like that, but Take 1 performed very well and produced an excellent impression, particularly with the combination that I described above. Give Take 1 a try. Order from your dealer or call Kerr at (800) KERR 123.

Pearl 113

Position Penta Impression Material
by 3M ESPE

When 3M ESPE introduced the unique Pentamix automix machine a few years ago, we assumed that this fancy machine was great for Impregum. But what if you used some other impression material? 3M ESPE proved us all wrong by introducing a full line of impression materials that is mixed by the very

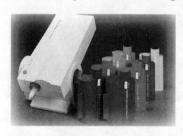

efficient and consistent Pentamix. The latest in this line of impression materials is a silicone product that has been formulated to replace alginate. I have been using this material for about three months in the office and have found it to be great for preliminary impressions and study-model impressions. This product is automatically mixed, stable, elastic, durable, and can be disinfected. The resulting impressions have better detail than alginates, and they are unaffected by evaporation, temperature, and humidity. Using the Pentamix to automatically mix the material, you will eliminate the dust, messy mixing bowls, and the wasted time and materials associated with alginate impressions. Since the Position Penta has the accuracy and elasticity of a PVS impression, you can pour these impressions multiple times with outstanding tear resistance. This could truly replace alginate in your office. To order, call your dealer, or for more information, check them out on the web at www.espeusa.com.

Pearl 114

Imprint II
Quick Step HB/LB
Impression Material
by 3M ESPE

If you are looking for a quick-set impression material with all the great accuracy of a long-set material, then try this material from 3M ESPE. Quick Step has been specially for-mulated to give you quick results while using a triple tray. You save time and material with this type of impression technique. This is meant for those quick procedures like single crowns or a couple of inlays. You have 40 sec-onds of intraoral working time and a two-and-a-half-minute setting time.

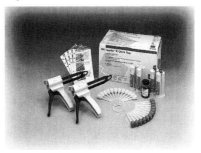

All this with excellent tear strength and terrific detail production. I have some more good news: the Quick Step cartridges will fit the reg-ular 3M ESPE dispenser, type HP. I have had problems in the past with the consistency of fast-set impression materials. This is one you can count on to have excellent results every time you use it. After using both heavy-bodied and light-bodied on a number of impressions, I pre-fer the light-bodied wash material. Call 3M ESPE at (800) 634-2249 or visit www.3M.com/dental.

Pearl 115

Imprint II SBR Occlusal Registration Material
by 3M ESPE

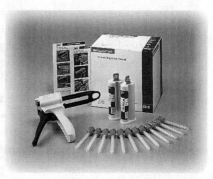

This material is an addition to the popular Imprint II line of impression materials. You will need the 3M ESPE Type HP dispenser to use this material, so be sure you have one of these before you order. As I told you before, be prepared for a wholesale changeover in the dispensing guns for cartridge-type materials. The material does a great job of getting a fast, accurate, and rigid interocclusal record. It resists slumping and offers very minimal resistance to closure, assuring a proper occlusal record. You have a 30-second working time and a one-minute set time in the mouth. You or the laboratory can easily trim the material. This is an all-around good material that is a great addition to the Imprint II line. Order from your dealer.

$\mathcal{P}earl$ 116

Easy Tray
by the Easy Tray Company

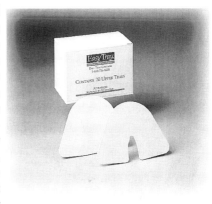

This product has been around for a while, and I am sure that a lot of dentists already are using it, but I just "discovered" it as I was walking through the exhibits at the California Dental Association meeting in Anaheim. I usually have avoided custom impression trays because of all the steps and stinky materials involved in making them. When I need one, I send it off to the lab to have it fabricated, and that gets expensive. This Easy Tray material has greatly simplified the process of making custom trays. The process was invented and is marketed by a dentist, Dr. John Wagner, and his wife, Nancy, out of Seattle. This new tray is not an acrylic, so there is no mixing, no smell, no liquids spilling, and no mess! This is a thermoplastic material that is supplied in the shape of upper and lower base plates. It is made moldable by placing it in water over 190 degrees for about 15 seconds. The water can be boiling, and you can leave the material in the water for hours with no change — it just stays soft. Amazing! Or, you can soften it in a bowl of water and zap it in the microwave for a couple of minutes. Unlike acrylic, you are not racing a set time, so you can start and stop during the construction of the tray. You can reuse the excess. I make most of my trays in the mouth using a disposable fluoride tray for a spacer. It is quick and easy, and the tray is ready in less than one minute. I can make a full-arch tray or just cut the amount I need to make a quadrant tray. I mold the material in the mouth and then remove it and cool it under cold tap water. Dry the tray and paint it with your usual tray adhesive. It is comfortable for the patients, and I use

• •

about one-third to one-half as much impression material as I do with a stock rim-lock tray. And, we don't have to worry about getting the trays back from the lab and cleaning and sterilizing them. Wow! That really saves some time and eliminates a messy job for the dental assistants. You could do the trays on a model, but that requires a lot more steps. John and Nancy also make a denture-base plate material called Easy Base, which is thinner and works the same way. This is a "no brainer"! Try it; I am confident that you will love the results. Order from your dealer or call Kerr or Easy Tray Company at (800) KERR-123.

Pearl 117

SureLoc
by Van R Dental Products

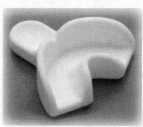

When I use disposable impression trays, usually the impression material pulls away from the tray, no matter how many holes or how much adhesive I put on. To solve this problem, Van R has come up with a nifty disposable impression tray system called SureLoc. It is a rigid tray that also has a porous quality, which bonds any impression material with a mechanical lock. SureLoc's rigid construction gives you an optimum seating compression of a nonperforated tray, yet you can easily and quickly trim it with a blade or a lab carbide for a truly custom fit. It has a nice anatomical design that requires little advanced trimming for patient comfort. SureLoc eliminates the need for any messy tray adhesive. The only problem is that a full-arch tray is not available. The impression tray comes in a half-arch left, half-arch right, and anterior sizes. Order from your dealer. For details, call Van R Dental Products at (800) 833-8267 or visit www.vanr.com.

$\mathcal{P}earl$ *118*

Quad Impression Tray
by Clinician's Choice

I have been using this quadrant impression tray for more than two years now, but I forgot to tell you about it. The Quad tray is a disposable, metal-framed "triple" tray, meaning that the opposing teeth are impressed at the same time as the prepped teeth in a closed bite impression technique. The metal frame, when combined with one of the new heavy-bodied impression materials, gives you a finished impression that is much more ridged than the plastic trays. Distortion is the biggest

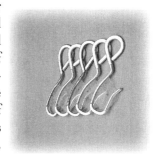

drawback of this impression technique. Your lab will like this because there is less likelihood of distortion as the impression is poured and mounted. This tray has a thinned-out piece of metal that spans facial lingual in the most posterior part. It is important to try this tray while empty to be certain that this posterior strip of metal does not impinge on tooth or tissue. This could cause the tray to distort. Of course, empty tray try-in should be part of your standard routine before any impression. This is a great impression tray that I could not practice without. Thanks, Peter, for another nifty product. Order from Clinician's Choice at (800) 265-3444.

Pearl 119

Three-Way Trays
by Sultan Dental Products

I f you are using triple trays in your impression or bite-registration techniques, give Sultan's new Three-Way Trays a try. They come in Anterior, Posterior, Quadrant, and, my favorite, the "Sideless." The

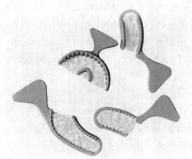

plastic frames are more rigid than most, so this should improve the accuracy of your impressions. Sultan has incorporated a nifty feature into its trays—an identification label is attached permanently to the tray handle so the impression will not get lost at the lab. Call your dealer to order Sultan's Three-Way Trays.

$\mathcal{P}earl$ *120*

Kromopan 100
by Kromopan USA

This is the original color-change alginate. There are many imitators on the market, but this is the best, in my opinion. The colors are very definite, and I know that when the material is white, I can seat the tray and the material 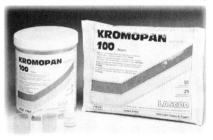 sets in about 30 seconds. My patients love it—no more gagging! Each phase of the procedure (spatulate, load tray, and insert in the mouth) is signaled clearly by a change in color. You have a perfect impression every time, with great detail and dimensional stability, and a happy patient. Call Kromopan USA at (847) 298-1259 or (800) 841-7398 to order.

Pearl 121

The Alginator
by Cadco

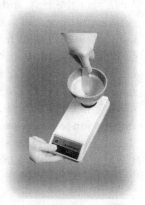

This is like a Mixmaster for your alginate impressions. It takes the problems out of mixing alginate and provides a mix that is bubble-free, simple, predictable, and consistent. This electric mixer spins a plastic bowl so that all you have to do is hold the spatula against the side of the bowl to mix the material. Everyone in the office loves using it; we would not mix alginate any other way. We have been using The Alginator for about 20 years and are on our second one, which is about 10 years old. It just keeps on mixing—the only thing we buy is an occasional new bowl. You get a smooth mix every time, and the mixer helps pick up the alginate and load the tray. When you hand-mix alginate, you trap air each time you fold the material on itself. The mixer eliminates bubbles and gives you error-free impressions. Your alginate will be very smooth, no matter what brand you use. My favorite, Kromopan, mixes very well in it. Cleanup is quick and easy if you follow the directions and pretreat the mixing bowl with a special spray. Another messy job has been automated and made quick and easy. Order from your dealer.

$\mathcal{P}earl$ *122*

Jumbo Syringe System
by Centrix

T he people at Centrix have come up with a great one this time. Now, there is finally a syringe on the market that's ideal for those viscous, hard-to-squeeze impression materials like Polygel, Impregum, and other monophase for-mulas. The disposable Jumbo tube and plug cartridge holds up to seven times the volume of the standard needle tubes. That is about 1.5 mil-liliters of material. This allows you to syringe precisely around several teeth. The 18-gauge needle tip reaches deep down into the sulcus to reduce voids and capture the finest details. Another plus is no more tired hands. A new leverage design allows you to place extremely thick and viscous materials without strain and hand-cramping. The Jumbo tube is easy to 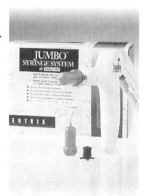 load. It can be backloaded off a mixing pad, directly from a Pentamix unit or from an automix cartridge. The tube and plug are fully dispos-able, so you eliminate cleanups and cross-contamination. This is defi-nitely a big timesaver. Call Centrix direct at (800) 235-5862 to order or for more information.

Chapter Eight

Cements

Pearl 123

RecyXVLC
(Vitremer Luting Cement)
by 3M Dental Products

I have been searching for the ideal cement since I began doing crowns and bridges—that one cement that I can use for everything. Well, guess what? It does not exist. However, if you are looking for a cement that is easy to use for porcelain-fused-to-metal crowns and all-metal inlays and crowns, then I

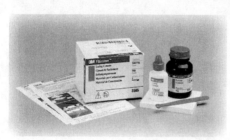

urge you to try RecyXVLC. Formerly known as Vitremer Luting Cement, this material is a major breakthrough in dental-cement technology. Vitremer is a glass ionomer resin that combines the best characteristics of both materials into one. You get all the great properties of a glass ionomer combined with the important resin cement advantages of zero solubility and high-fracture toughness. Zero solubility provides high confidence in marginal integrity, whereas fracture toughness provides increased confidence in the cement performance. Vitremer Luting Cement chemically bonds to tooth structure without acid-etch techniques, releases fluoride, has a moderate strength that allows for later crown removal, and is radiopaque. When mixed, the material takes on a mousse-like consistency, which makes it easy to pick up with an instrument. This lack of flow does require some practice when loading the crown. Your assistants will love the ease of mixing, loading, and cleanup of instruments. No more scraping set cement off the instruments. Cleanup of excess cement is very quick and easy a few minutes after seating the crown. Since I have been using Vitremer Luting Cement,

• •

reports of tooth sensitivity while seating and reports of postoperative tooth sensitivity have been almost zero. So there you have it…a cement with all the properties you are looking for—chemical bond; fluoride release; strength; zero solubility; easy to mix, load, seat, and clean up; and no sensitivity. Order from your dealer.

Pearl 124

Fuji Plus Capsules
by GC America

Thanks to GC, we now have a resin-reinforced, glass-ionomer cement in a capsule for easy, consistent mixes. It is easy to use, with remarkable strength, sustained fluoride release, and excellent biocompatibility. Fuji Plus bonds to metal and porcelain-fused-to-metal crowns and bridges, inlays, and onlays. It also bonds to all types of core build-up material. It bonds chemically to the tooth with a significant, long-term fluoride release. This cement is great because of the low film thickness it exhibits. The bond strengths are higher than other comparable cements. This is a cement that sets quickly, too. In about 30 seconds, the material is in a rubbery stage, ready to be removed. Fuji Plus gives you a quick and easy cementing technique. The cement is a translucent color for good blending with tooth structure. Give it a try. I think you will like it. Order from your dealer or call GC America for more information at (800) 323-7063.

$\mathcal{P}earl$ 125

PermaCem
by Zenith

This product is a compomer-based cement. These resin-reinforced glass ionomer permanent cements can be used for the final cementation of all metal crowns and inlays, porcelain-fused-to-metal crowns and bridges, and crowns with aluminous cores. PermaCem is self-curing, radiopaque, and releases fluoride. It handles well, like most other

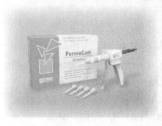

cements of this type, and cleans up easily. The fascinating part about PermaCem is the automix delivery system. You quickly get a consistent, homogenous mix that is easy to put wherever you want it. No messy tubes, no variances in amounts of material, no hand mixing, no pads...this is too easy! Just pick up the dispensing gun, pull the trigger,

and instantly you have a perfectly mixed cement in your crown ready to seat with no waiting. The cement will set to a rubbery stage in less than two minutes. This is the time to clean off the excess. If you leave your patient or wait too long, the cement sets quite hard, and you will have a difficult time removing the excess. So follow the directions carefully, and you really will like this cement. I feel that you will waste less material than hand mixing, because you only use as much as you need. Please remember, this cement contains glass ionomer that expands; do not use with ceramic restorations. PermaCem is dispensed from the same Type-25 applicator gun that is used for Luxacore and Tempocem. I think this is a great product that will make your cementation appointment faster, easier, and better. Order from your dealer or call Zenith at (800) 662-6383.

$\mathscr{P}earl\ 126$

Rely X ARC Adhesive Resin Cement
by 3M ESPE

The 3M ESPE company is doing some name changing. The family of 3M ESPE cements will now be known by the general brand name of Rely X. Rely X ARC is a permanent, dual-cure resin cement to be used for the final cementation of crowns, bridges, all-ceramic porcelain or composite crowns, bridges, inlays and onlays, and endodontic posts. I have found this to be an extreme-ly easy cement to work with. This is a paste-to-paste system that is quickly and easily dispensed onto a mixing pad using the clicker. The material is then spatulated to a creamy mix. Rely X ARC is compatible with one-bottle bond-

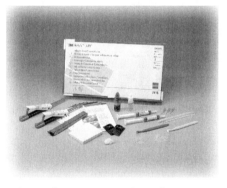

ing agents. The material will set in about five minutes, but the excess can be cleaned up in about three minutes when the material begins to "gel." The excess material will clean up very easily with a flick of an explorer. To save time, I usually remove the excess cement immediate-ly after seating the crown with a Microbrush. I carefully floss to remove interproximal excess and then light-cure for about 10 seconds on the facial and 10 seconds on the lingual. This will harden material at the gingival margin. Be sure to cure the margins after cleaning the excess. The material comes in an A1 transparent shade and shade A3. I think that 3M ESPE has a real winner here—a terrific resin cement and a great new dispensing system. Order from your dealer or call 3M ESPE at (800) 634-2249.

Pearl 127

Panavia 21
by J. Morita

I was just reintroduced to Panavia at the ADA show in Washington, DC. I quit using Panavia as a cement years ago, because it was so messy and inconsistent. Now I find that there is new packaging and 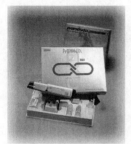 formulation that make using it extremely simple. If you have had a similar experience, you may want to take another look at the Panavia cement. The new paste-to-paste formulation provides a consistent mix with exact setting times every time you use it. A twist of the knob on the new package dispenses a precise amount of paste for mixing. It's great for bonding metal, silanated porcelain, composite, and amalgam. Call J. Morita at (800) 752-9729 for additional information on Panavia 21 or to place your order.

$\mathcal{P}earl$ *128*

Compolute Aplicap
by ESPE

Now we have a dual-cure, composite-resin cement in the convenience of a capsule. I have been using Compolute for my inlays and veneers with great results. The capsule mixing gives me a consistency of mix and an ease of handling and delivery. The material has a medium viscosity that does not run or slump when placed, but it has a very low film thickness that allows you to fully seat your restorations. The applicator allows for simple, direct placement of the material onto the tooth or into the restoration. Since the mix is controlled, the setting time is exact with every patient. Using a throw-away capsule enhances our infection-control system and saves time on cleanup. The material comes in four great shades. I particularly like the inclusion of a chameleon or neutral shade, so that the cement does not affect the shade of my finished restoration. It comes with a great bonding system as well. Thanks, ESPE, for another terrific product! Order from your dealer or call ESPE at (800) 344-8235.

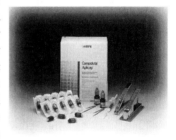

$\mathscr{P}earl$ 129

Nexus Universal Luting System
by Kerr

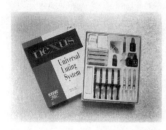

T his system replaces Kerr's aging Porcelite luting system. When I first looked at this system in Chicago last year, I was skeptical. I wanted to know how three shades would be enough to handle all situations. I have been using the Nexus system for about three months now and guess what? Three shades are great! The kit contains everything you need to bond porcelain: great try-in pastes that easily clean up with water; resin cement, loaded in syringes, for easy dispensing and little waste; the resin cement can be dual- or light-cure, depending on the situation; the resin cement is thicker than Porcelite (a great improvement), so it has a better viscosity; the cement contains fluoride; and the bonding agents are enclosed. With the resin packed in a syringe, you can dispense directly to the veneer or crown and have no waste. The steps for bonding are easy and quick. If you are doing six anterior veneers, you can apply the bond to all the teeth and then follow right up with the resin-filled veneers. The Nexus system makes porcelain bonding much easier. Call Kerr at (800) KERR-123 for additional information or order the Nexus Universal Luting system from your dealer. Update: This system has been replaced by the new and improved Nexus 2 Luting System.

$\mathscr{P}earl\ 130$

Calibra
by Dentsply/Caulk

This is a esthetic resin cement from Dentsply Caulk. I am excited about it, because it can be used for crowns, bridges, inlays and onlays, and veneers. Calibra comes in a five-shade base system that is light-curable. Also included are a regular-viscosity and a high-viscosity color-stable catalyst for dual-cure capability when you need it. This material uses the proven Prime & Bond NT bonding system in either a light-cure or a dual-cure system. The proven simplicity of the Prime & Bond NT two-bottle dual-cure system takes out all the guesswork. It dispenses and mixes easily and is easy to load into the veneers and crowns. This is a complete system that satisfies all esthetic needs. The Operatory Kit (one syringe of translucent base and one syringe of light-shade base) comes close to what I requested from Caulk. Perhaps someday we will be able to buy a kit of three or four syringes of translucent base with a couple of syringes of catalyst. Then we will have a kit to cement veneers without changing the shade that we have ordered from the lab. Call your dealer to order Calibra.

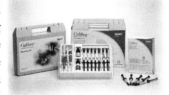

$\mathcal{P}earl$ *131*

Encore Solo and ProxiDiscs
by Centrix

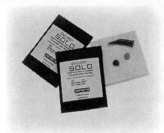

Here are two great products that will make your life easier in the treatment room. Encore Solo is a light-cure composite core paste for no-mix core buildups. It comes packaged in prefilled syringe tubes so that you can go directly from package to mouth without cross-contamination. Use it once and then dispose of it. This material comes out of the tube in a translucent blue color that changes to pink to indicate complete polymerization. What a great idea! The material cures quickly and deeply. It releases fluoride, has good resistance to cutting with a diamond, and is compatible with all light-cure composite bonding agents. Try this one; I know you will like it. The second product from Centrix is so simple that you will wonder why someone did not think of it sooner. If you are doing any anterior cosmetic work, you must have the ProxiDisc. No matter how careful you are, you will bond two teeth together during a cosmetic procedure. When that happens, I try floss, strips, whatever to break the bond, and it usually takes longer than I like! Now you have the ProxiDisc as a solution to that problem. They are amazingly thin stainless-steel discs that are an indispensable tool in any dental practice. You simply roll the ProxiDisc through the interproximal area with minimal pressure to remove polymerized bonding agents and other hard-to-remove materials. They are much safer than a sharp instrument and are certainly more reliable and easier to use than floss or strips. ProxiDiscs are manufactured with a hole in the handle to allow tying of a safety loop of dental floss. They are sterilizable by any method and are available with smooth or sandblasted (abrasive) sides. This is a must-have product! Order it today by calling Centrix at (800) 235-5862 or fax (888) CENTRIX.

$\mathcal{P}earl$ *132*

Provilink
by Vivadent

Have you been looking for a temporary cement that sets quick-ly, is eugenol-free, cleans up easily, removes easily, and leaves no residue on the tooth? Well, look no more. Provilink is your answer. This material is amazing. It mixes easily, with no smearing or sticking when you lute your tempo-rary crowns and bridges. Then, you simply seat the temps and light-cure for 10 to 20 seconds on the margins, and the excess can be removed immediately. The material is dual-curing, which assures thor-

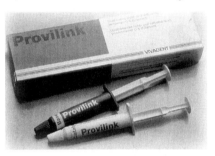

ough polymerization of the entire restoration. It has an antibacterial effect and a fluoride release. Our patients have reported reduced sensi-tivity since we began using this material. When you remove the tempo-rary crown, the material does not stick to the tooth, so you eliminate the need to clean temporary cement off the tooth. Wow! What a great time-saver! Order from your dealer.

●●●●●●●●●●●●●●●●●●●●●●●●

Pearl 133

TempBond™ Clear
by Kerr

Y ou all are familiar with TempBond™ temporary cement. It comes in a couple of tubes, and you mix them together and get a white temporary cement. TempBond™ Clear is a dual-cure, resin-based temporary cement for use in cementing temporary and provisional restorations like crowns, bridges, veneers, inlays, and onlays. When cured, the material is transparent. It does not change the shade of the beautiful temporaries that you made. No more white spots or cement show-through, so you get better esthetics. 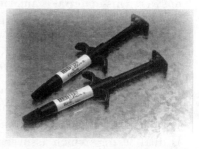 Since it is dual-cure, you can hit the material with your curing light and begin cleanup knowing that you will also get a chemical cure. Wait! There's more. The material remains flexible after setting, so cleanup is very easy—the excess just peels off. I have found that I get a good seal, no sensitivity, and good retention. There's more good news: the temps are easy to remove and the material cleans up very simply, so you are ready to try on and cement your permanent restoration. The exceptional handling, ease of mix, and easy cleanup make TempBond™ Clear my choice for a temporary cement. Order from your dealer or call Kerr at (800) KERR-123.

$\mathcal{P}earl$ *134*

True-Grip
by Clinician's Choice

True-Grip tips are three inches long and have an adhesive tip that
is ideal for handling veneers,
crowns, bridges, posts, inlays,
and onlays. They will easily and tena-
ciously adhere to any small item with
just a touch, making movement from
the operative tray to the mouth easy
and effective. This certainly minimizes
the chance of dropping or damaging
the item. The tips are bendable and can
be reused for multiple units. To order,
call (800) 265-3444. Thanks to Peter
Jordan for another great product.

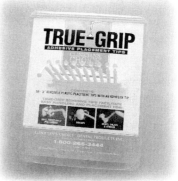

Chapter Nine

Dentures

$\mathcal{P}earl$ 135

Predictable Complete Dentures
by Dr. Joseph J. Massad

If you have problems getting consistent results on your complete-denture patients, then this is for you. I quit doing dentures many years ago because I could not get consistent results. Then implants came along, and I was doing dentures again. I needed help, so I went to one of Dr. Joe Massad's seminars. He presented an extremely organized procedure for producing a predictable complete denture. Now he has put the technique on video. This two-tape series carries his lecture to a new level of excellence. This is a professionally done, well-edited video that presents Dr. Massad treating a patient in his office. The step-by-step presentation is easy to understand and follow. If you want to begin getting consistent results with your complete-denture patients, order this videotape. It is, without a doubt, the very best complete-denture course that I have ever seen! Dr. Massad covers everything from the patient exam all the way through the denture delivery. For additional information or to place your order, call (800) 800-3115 and ask for extension DE.

$\mathcal{P}earl$ *136*

Dr. Joseph Massad Denture Kit
by Brasseler USA

My good friend, Dr. Joe Massad, has put together a wonderful kit that provides all the acrylic and soft-liner cutters that you need for making adjustments to dentures. If you have taken Joe's course or have his fantastic video, "Predictable Complete

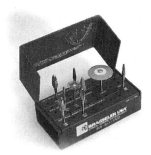

Dentures," you need this kit to easily do the adjustments that he recommends. The kit comes with instructions for each bur and polisher permanently etched in the top of the bur holder. You will not forget what each one is for, and the reorder numbers are also permanently etched. By following the principles outlined in Dr. Massad's courses and his video (available through Dental Economics), you can develop a technique that will enable you to deliver dentures that fit with a consistency that you never thought possible. For additional information or to order your kit, call Brasseler USA at (800) 841-4522.

$\mathcal{P}earl$ *137*

Multi-Cup Dentures
by Aesthetic Porcelain Studios

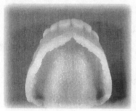

D o you watch the nightly news on one of the major networks? Do you pay attention to who the major advertisers of these programs are? Night after night on these national news programs, we are bombarded by commercials for denture adhesives. Do you think that this may be an indication that loose dentures are a problem in the United States? If so, you are right! There are 43,000,000 people in the U.S. who are edentulous or partially edentulous. The basic concern of these people is getting dentures that "fit." What they really want is RETENTION! What if you could give it to them? Would this be a new market for your practice? You can, by using Multi-Cup dentures that actually have many tiny suction cups contacting the tissue and holding the denture in place. Dentists across the country have discovered this technology and are attracting many new patients to their practices. Actually, the original patent for suction cup dentures goes back over a hundred years, but in the last 20 years the technique has been developed and enhanced by Dr. Arthur Jermyn. He has developed a system and technique for the production of suction cups onto a soft silicone denture liner. Labs have been slow to pick up the technique because it is not simple enough. About eight years ago, my good friend David Block began experimenting with polymers, silicone, suction-cup design, and angulation, and he perfected a fantastic product for labs, dentists, and patients-truly a win/win/win situation. This baby really sticks! The suction cups comfortably latch onto the tissue and really provide goop-free retention. David refers to it as the "Octopus" denture. So if you want to get in on this great market, give David a call at (800) 544-9605 for more information.

$\mathscr{P}earl$ 138

Tokuso Rebase
by Tokuyama

This product represents a breakthrough in hard chairside relining. This material and the accompanying technique allow you to achieve a tight, accurate fit while the rebase cures in the mouth. There is no methyl methacrylate for you or the patient to deal with. A newly developed acrylic monomer cures without heat or chemical irritation, so you can do a true in-the-mouth chairside reline, and the patient won't hate you for it. In the past few years, the light-cure reline materials have been highly touted, but these materials are composites and do not adhere well to the acrylic denture base. Tokuso Rebase supplies a "Rebase AID," which enhances the bond between the

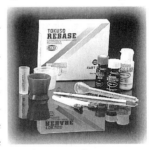

resin and the denture base. It is easy to mix, and the fine powder ensures good flow characteristics. So, if you want faster, better, and easier chairside full-denture relines, try Tokuso Rebase. Since people are keeping their teeth longer than ever, many dentists are doing a lot more partial dentures. About six or seven years after the partial is made, it needs to be relined. Probably the best material to use, because of its great flow, is the Tokuso Rebase. You will find that the material has a great color stability. It definitely is the best of the chairside rebase materials. The lack of methyl methacrylate and the very low heat-setting reaction beat out all similar products. If you have a problem getting reline materials to adhere to the surface of nonprecious metals, such as metal-palate dentures, try Mr. Bond from Tokuso. It gives a strong adhesion between the rebase and the nonprecious metal, is easy to use, and will give you a very durable reline. Run, don't walk, to the phone and order Tokuso Rebase and Mr. Bond, or call Tokuyama at (800) 275-2867.

$\mathscr{P}earl$ *139*

SoftLine
by Micro Select

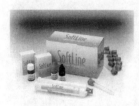

This is a new chairside silicone soft-relining system that is applied chairside via an auto-mix cartridge delivery system. The Soft-Line material is easy to use, has a good consistency that will stay where you put it, is not runny, and sets in the mouth in three minutes or less. SoftLine can be used to relieve pressure areas, provide post damming in the case of adhesion problems, and for cushioning of implants when using an overdenture during the healing process. The bonding agent provided achieves a very strong bond with denture acrylic. SoftLine trims easily and polishes quickly with a varnish material to smooth trimmed borders. Micro Select is a division of MicroDental Laboratories. Call (800) 840-2650 for more information or to order.

$\mathscr{P}earl$ 140

The Soft Relining System
by Tokuyama

C hairside soft relines were never so quick and simple as this. An automix cartridge system delivers bubble-free resin in one easy step. This material is a silicone-based resin that elimi- nates offensive odors, heat irrita- tion, and unpleasant taste while it cures entirely in the mouth. The use of silicone in the material decreases stains and odors. The manufacturer claims that a new adhesive primer strengthens the bonding between the resin and

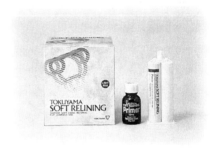

the denture for a longer-lasting reline. I have been using this system for about six months now and find it to be superior to other chairside soft-reline systems. Give it a try. Order from your dealer or call Tokuyama at (800) 275-2867.

Pearl 141

PermaSoft® Soft Denture Liner
by Austenal

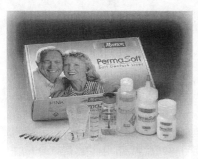

T his unique product is an intermediate to long-term chairside soft-liner for dentures. Most soft-liners on the market are meant for short-term use. You know the scenario; the patient comes back in six to eight weeks and the material stinks and is pulling away from the denture. PermaSoft is different! First, it is the only methyl-methacrylate-free soft-liner on the market. So you don't have to deal with a pungent odor and possible sensitivity problems. It is an extremely easy product to use. Simply mix the proper amount of powder and liquid to the correct viscosity and place it into a clean denture that has been roughened. Place it in the mouth, muscle trim, and allow to set. You then remove the denture and finish the cure in hot water for only 15 minutes. At this point, the most important step is to dry the denture and apply two coats of sealer, following directions. If you need to adjust, the material will bond to itself. The PermaSoft bonds chemically to the denture without a special bonding agent. The amazing thing is that the bond to the denture is long-lasting, and the material remains soft. It is recommended that you reseal the denture on an annual basis. I think you will find that PermaSoft will take care of many of your problem denture patients. To order, call Austenal at (800) 621-0381.

$\mathcal{P}earl\ 142$

Dinabase®
by Sultan Chemists

Dinabase is a single-component, no-mix thermoplastic material that is used for long-term tissue conditioning, temporary relining, and functional impressions. The material is directly applied with a dispenser syringe that makes for a fast, easy application. The material cartridge is softened in hot water. Dinabase has no odor and no heat; it adheres to acrylic resin without bonding agents; and it is non-sticking and nontoxic. Setup and cleanup times are incredibly fast. Upon setting, Dinabase is easy to trim, and it produces a great impression. At any point during the procedure, you can add to the material or correct a void by reheating the material. Final finishing is accomplished 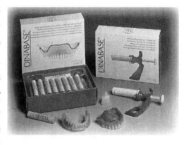 by heating the material in the denture and reseating it. Dinabase is a product that really fits the faster, easier, and better model. Order from your dealer or call Sultan Chemists at (800) 637-8582.

$\mathcal{P}$earl 143

Carbide Lab Burs
by Brasseler USA

For my money, Brasseler has some of the best-cutting burs for acrylics, alloys, plaster, and castings. If you want to adjust, reduce, cut, or shape, they probably have an instrument for it. The company has just brought out two terrific burs. One of the worst jobs in the dental office is to remove an old chairside soft liner from a denture. The

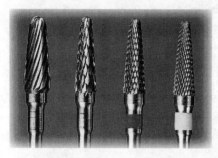 material stinks, and it is hard to remove. Now comes a cutter designed just for this job. Brasseler has nicknamed it the "Terminator." It is a wicked-looking cutter, but it really does the job. In a quarter of the time it usually takes me, I was able to quickly and easily remove the soft liner. Every one of you needs one of these in the lab. Your assistants will bless you. Ask for the Terminator or the SG-Cutter Blade. Another problem that I have is trimming soft reline material, particularly the lab-processed materials. Most cutters just bounce off of the material, so adjustments to it are a pain. Well, Brasseler has solved that problem, too, by designing a cutter to trim soft reline material and mouthguard material. If you do soft relines or mouthguards, you need this instrument. Ask for the FSQ-Straight-Bladed Cutter. Call Brasseler USA at (800) 841-4522 for more information.

●   ●

$\mathscr{P}earl$ *144*

System2
by Accu-Dent Research and Development Company

Do you have problems with the fit of your partial dentures? Do you take a preliminary impression and make a custom try for your final? Do you agree that the secret to great-fitting partials is a great impression? If you have answered "yes" to any of these questions, I can save you some time and aggravation. The folks at Accu-Dent have been around since 1970 with what they call a "Multi-Colloid" concept. You may have tried it at one time or another like I did and had mixed results. Forget the past. Accu-Dent has a great product with its System2. The system utilizes new, anatomically designed impression trays that really work. Accu-Dent's Multi-Colloid

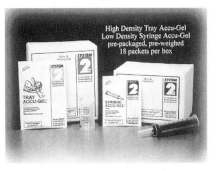

impression technique uses two different irreversible hydrocolloids in a single-entry impression. The light-bodied Syringe Gel is applied to the teeth under hydraulic pressure, with a unique syringe system to eliminate air bubbles, and to the vestibules for border-molding. The heavy-bodied Tray Gel is brought to the mouth directly after the application of the Syringe Gel. The tray gel further pressurizes the syringe gel around the teeth, places absolutely uniform pressure over the edentulous ridge areas, and will not flow down the patient's throat. The two materials merge into a single, high-quality impression, with no bubbles, excellent border-molding and great detail. Since Accu-Dent recommends 80- to 85-degree water for mixing, your patient will be very comfortable. The total time for upper and lower impressions is less than 15 minutes. So, let's recap what we have here: a final impression on the first appointment, a total time of less than eight minutes per impression, at a cost of less than two bucks per impression, with easy cleanup, with very good patient comfort and tolerance and, last but not least, great-fitting partials. Looks like a no-brainer to me! You save at least one appointment, have no remakes, and the material costs less. A video comes with the system, and Accu-Dent has a 60-day "Try it in your own operatory" guarantee. Call Accu-Dent Research and Development Company at (800) 344-5457 for information on ordering or a lab near you that is familiar with the System2.

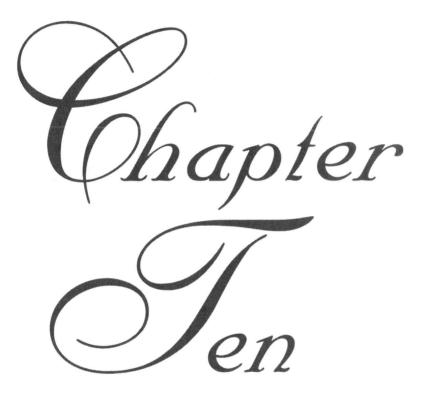

Chapter Ten

Prophy, Sealants

$\mathcal{P}earl\ 145$

JetShield
by DENTSPLY Preventive Care

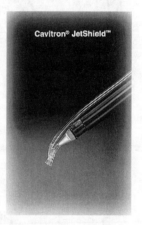

Cavitron® JetShield™

Does your hygienist use a Prophy Jet? Do you want to buy her something she will thank you for every time she uses it? If so, buy her the new JetShield. This is a simple device that works! Attach the disposable tubing to the tip of the Prophy Jet and attach the other end either to the suction system or to the saliva-ejection system. Now there is a cup-shaped device at the end of the Prophy Jet that fits snugly against the tooth that evacuates the aerosols produced. Spray and splatter are reduced by 97 percent. My hygienists always have liked the Prophy Jet, but have complained about the spray. Over the years, most hygienists learn to control the spray, but it always has been a problem. They put up with the inconvenience of the spray because they have always felt that air polishing does a better job of removing stains, plaque, and soft debris. Our patients like the fresh, minty feel in their mouths after we are finished. JetShield's design ensures that you are working at the proper angulation and distance from the tooth. Combine this with the virtual elimination of spray, and the results are greater patient comfort and greater visibility when you are working. You also can use the tip to eliminate any saliva that may be pooling elsewhere in the mouth. It is very convenient. Once you have completed a procedure, simply dispose of the used Jet-Shield. This is a no-brainer! Order now from your local dealer or call DENTSPLY Preventive Care at (800) 989-8826 for more information.

$\mathscr{P}earl$ *146*

Pro-Select 3 System
by Pro-Dentec

T his product is a piezo-ultrasonic scaler/irrigation system that incorporates everything the dentist and hygienist have been asking for in this type of instrument. The entire handpiece, the tips, the cables, and the bottles are fully auto-clavable. There are no more compromises in your infection-control system and no more wrapping cables—just put everything in the autoclave. If you have used the piezo-electric systems, you know how quiet they are for operator and patient. Since the Pro-Select 3 System is a closed, multifluid system for scaling and irrigation, the concerns about biofilm are eliminated. The system offers three new, interchangeable tips—right, universal, and left Ultraslim tips—which provide all the versatility you will need. My hygienist is able to do more in less time and with less fatigue using the piezo-ultrasonic system. Another great plus for this product is that you control all functions with the multifunctional foot control. There is no need to return constantly to the control unit to make changes; the foot control does it all. The cable connections for this new system are very simple. There are no plugs to line up—just a simple snap on and off. The irrigator handpiece will warm the medicaments for sub-gingival irrigation, so there's no more sensitivity when you want to irrigate. You can elect to scale with purified water or with medicaments; it's your choice! This is a great product from a great company that stands behind its products with terrific, after-the-sale customer service. Your hygienist will love you! Call Pro-Dentec at (800) 752-2565 to order.

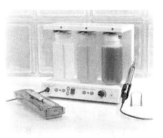

Pearl 147

Implant-Prophy+
by AIT Dental, Inc.

T his is a plastic dental-instrument system designed for safe and effective debridement of implants, root-sensitive areas, and around composites and veneers. The instruments come in standard dimensions and blade angles such as Gracey 5/6, 11/12, 13/14, and Columbia 13/14U. One of my problems with this type of instru-

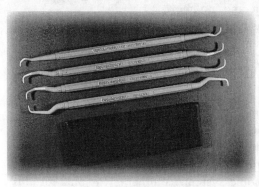

ment is feeling that I am removing debris, but these instruments have exceptional sharpness and strength. You can resharpen them many times with a special stone that is included with the instruments. They are autoclavable and certified as FDA Class 3 devices, so they are in full compliance with regulatory protocol. If you have been looking for instruments to use around implants and with your beautiful cosmetic restorations, look no further. Call (800) 876-4620 for details or order from your dealer.

$\mathscr{P}earl$ *148*

Upgrade Prophy Angle
by Sultan

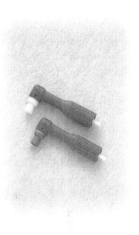

There really is not a whole lot new in prophy angles; in the past, I usually just bought the least expensive one I could find...until I tried Sultan's new Upgrade. This one is different. There is no more chatter or those "squirrelly" noises that aggravate you with most disposable angles. This one runs smoother longer than any angle I have tried. So, when you press a little harder to get rid of some stubborn stain, the angle does not give up and die. The cup is well-designed to control splatter of paste. Order from your dealer or call Sultan at (800) 238-6739.

● ●

$\mathcal{P}earl$ 149

Disposable Prophy Angle
by Prophy Perfect, Inc.

I know that most dentists have tried throw-away prophy angles and either liked them or hated them. If you like them, then this product is for you. These angles come with a natural rubber cup that will not heat up or break apart. This is a solidly built unit with a thick shell that eliminates vibration and heat-up. The gear system is very quiet and is double-lubricated to prevent freezing of the angle. The unit is guaranteed to last through the entire prophylaxis procedure, or the company will replace it free. I saved the best for last…the price is the best on the market! For more information or to order, call Prophy Perfect, Inc. at (800) 776-3948.

$\mathscr{P}earl$ 150

The Rota-dent
by Pro-Dentec

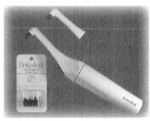

I have been dispensing this power brush in my practice since it first came out in 1985. The reason is simple. The results in all types of periodontal cases have been positive. Let's face it; most of our home-care programs have failed because of a lack of patient compliance. A home-care program with the Rota-dent is easier for the patient to follow, so I see better results more often. I like an office-dispensing program because I don't have to rely on the folks at Wal-Mart or Target to instruct my patients. I am able to monitor their progress, so I know they are using the power brush correctly. The Rota-dent is a power plaque-removing instrument that has been clinically proven to be equally effective to the combination of brushing, flossing, and interdental cleaning. There have been over 20 clinical articles published in leading dental journals. The instrument has a specially designed tip that reaches and cleans the areas below the gum and in between the teeth. In my practice, we have seen many patients able to control their periodontal disease and keep their teeth for a lifetime. Pro-Dentec has a professional staff on board to assist you, so give them a call at (800) 228-5595 for more information.

$\mathcal{P}earl$ 151

Proxi-Floss
by Advanced Implant Technologies

This is a disposable elastomeric appliance designed to clean interproximal spaces, bridges, implants, and orthodontic brackets and wires. This is a great product! It is easy to thread into spaces, under bridges, or implants, and it is the only cleaner that will hold together while cleaning ortho brackets and wires. It retains a full

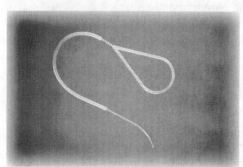

cleaning action under tension; it does not collapse like the fiber-based products do. It will not snag, fray, or shred. There is no metal or wires in the Proxi-Floss, so there is no galvanic shock and no traumatizing of the soft tissues. Proxi-Floss will carry medicaments to the mouth for precise delivery of chemotherapeutic agents. This is a great product for your patients. Order some today by calling (800) 876-4620 or order from your local dealer.

$\mathcal{P}earl$ 152

Delton FS+
by Dentsply Preventive Care

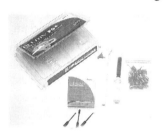

For many years, Delton has been a leader in pit-and-fissure sealants. Now an improved system offers a number of great features. Delton itself has changed and is now a 55 percent filled resin with fluoride that makes it a strong and wear-resistant sealant. In fact, you could call it a "flowable" resin. The resin material is packaged in the familiar Delton black with the long, bendable tip. But the end of the tip is new; a great "microbrush" is attached to it, allowing for better handling and movement of the sealant resin. You also can achieve total infection control with the new autoclavable applicator handle and the disposable sealant cartridges. The etchant syringe with a new microbrush tip ensures the etch gets into all the deep pits and fissures. Overall, this system makes sealing teeth faster, easier, and better. Order from your dealer. Call Dentsply Preventive Care for more information on Delton FS+ or visit their Web site at www.dentsply.com.

Pearl 153

The EcuSeal System
by Zenith Dental

EcuSeal is a sealant system. The delivery process is unique: the autoclavable Ecu-pen features a rolling mechanism that is at the operator's index finger to allow for easy, smooth, and accurate placement of both the EcuSeal and the Etch Gel. This dispensing

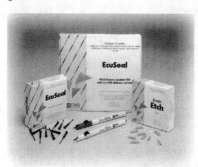

method is the key to the system. With it, you can easily control the flow and placement of the materials. EcuSeal is a light-cured, resin-based pit and fissure sealant, with a filler that releases fluoride and adds strength. Zinc has been added for its bacteriostatic qualities. It is packaged in a one-time-use, black Mikro-tip carpule that contains enough material to complete an entire quadrant of sealants. The blue Etch Gel is a 37 percent phosphoric acid packaged in a disposable, clear Mikro-tip carpule with enough for an entire quadrant. We (my hygienist and I) have used EcuSeal and have found the delivery system to make the application of a sealant quick and precise. I think you will like this system. It's faster, better, and easier! Order from your dealer or call Zenith Dental for more information at (800) 662-6383.

Pearl 154

Opalescence Tooth Whitening Family
by Ultradent

The folks at Ultradent have come up with a great combination of tooth-whitening products that cover all the bases. There is Opalescence 10 percent that comes in a number of flavors and is applied in a custom tray for daytime or overnight bleaching, which generally takes about one to two weeks to complete. The new Opalescence F comes in a 15 percent and a 20 percent carbamide peroxide formulation with fluoride release and a tasty melon flavor. Both of these products come in a sticky, thick gel that 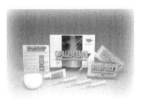 stays on the teeth where it belongs, and both have a 20 percent water content to minimize tooth dehydration. I recently bleached my teeth with the Opalescence F 20 percent and was able to finish the process in about five days. The material was easy to dispense and did not squeeze out of the tray or burn the tissue. I hate some of the flavors used in bleaching materials, but this one has a good taste. The other products in the group are Opalescence Quick, a 35 percent carbamide peroxide designed to be used at the dental office, but the patient sits in the waiting room rather than the operatory. Recommended treatment time is 30 minutes to two hours. Opalescence Xtra is a 35 percent hydrogen peroxide, chairside power bleach, which is light-activated. You can order everything you need for tooth-whitening from Ultradent, including Sof-Tray Sheets, LC Block-Out Resin, Pocket Tray Cases, a patient-education video, and marketing materials. For your sensitivity cases, use Flor-Opal, a sustained-release fluoride "sticky" gel designed to be used in the bleaching tray. It works great! Call (800) 552-5512 to place your order.

$\mathscr{P}earl$ 155

The Zaris™ Professional Tooth Whitening System
by 3M

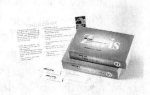

The innovative part of the Zaris™ system is in the fabrication of the bleaching trays. Without a doubt, the best way to start a bleaching case is to deliver the trays and bleach the same day that the patient decides to do it. But, most of the time, impressions are made, and the patient must return at a later date to receive the bleaching trays and begin treatment. The biggest problem has not been taking the impressions or pouring models, but painting the teeth with block-out resin and then curing the resin before making the bleaching tray. What if you could skip this step? 3M's Zaris™ System allows you to do just that. 3M has come up with a unique peel-and-stick gel retention insert that replaces time-consuming block-out resin. This material has a patented microreplicated surface to hold bleaching gel in the tray and against the teeth for faster results. So with new, fast-setting materials to pour the impressions with, the bleaching trays can be made in less than 15 minutes. The kits include easy-to-follow directions for quickly fabricating the bleaching trays. The trays were comfortable in my mouth, and the syringes of bleaching gel were easy to use. Everything you need is supplied in a convenient kit form. 3M has a convenient two-syringe touch-up kit to help patients maintain the great results. Also included are some great, free education materials. A clever smile-catching mirror is included so that patients can actually get a look at their teeth when no one else is looking. I liked the mint flavor of the gel and the good fit of the bleaching tray. If you are doing a lot of bleaching in the office, this could save you a lot of time in the process of making the trays. Faster, better, easier. To order, contact your authorized 3M™ Dental distributor. For more information, visit www.3M.com/dental or call (800) 634-2249.

$\mathscr{P}earl$ 156

Perfecta 3/15
by American Dental Hygienics

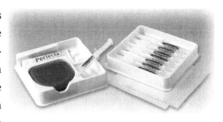

This is a new bleach that has just been brought on the market. We were introduced to it at the CDA meeting in Anaheim. Everyone at the office has tried and been delighted with the results. Now, you can have whitening in minutes, not hours. This revolutionary hydrogen peroxide gel requires only 15 minutes of wear time. With Perfecta 3/15, your patients will get the same or better results as with the traditional carbamide peroxide gels…in less time. Tooth-whitening has never been faster, easier, or more effective. And we have found that sensitivity is no longer a problem with this product. ADH has incorporated a buffering agent so that the material is dispensed at a pH of 7. It also is water-based, which causes less dehydration than other formulas. With short wear times two or three times a day, patient acceptance is better. Compliance is improved. The gel is very sticky so that it stays on the teeth where it will work. None of us had any tissue irritation or burning. Give this one a try! I think it will be the next generation of bleaching agents. To place your order, call American Dental Hygienics at (800) 832-7483.

𝒫earl 157

The Tidi Prophy and Knee-Length Bib
by Tidi Brand

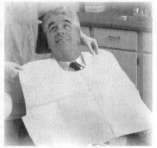

P robably no one knows who decided that the standard bib size should be 13" x 18", but that size hardly protects anybody from anything. I have seen stains on men's shirt collars and women's blouses more times than I would like to remember. I have tried several different approaches to avoid this. The beauty shop cover-up that attaches at the neck has problems, as it gets stained and dirty. The plastic cover-ups give your patients a steam bath while they are with you. Initially, nobody in the dental field could help. Nobody made a bib larger than 13" x 18". I looked over on the medical side and found several manufacturers that made large bibs for nursing homes that worked quite well. Then, Tidi came to dentistry with an oversized bib having a contour neck that provides full coverage through the shoulders and arms. The bib is a tissue-poly-tissue construction for moisture protection and to keep the bib from shifting on the patient. It provides ample coverage for any patient. Have you ever thought that a standard-size bib looked like a postage stamp on some people? The Tidi bib provides maximum coverage in the shoulder and neck areas. It comes in two sizes: the waist-length prophy bib at 29" x 21" that I use for hygiene and short operative appointments and the knee-length size at 29" x 42" that I use for all crown-and-bridge procedures. Protect your patients with a bib that really protects instead of the ridiculous 13" x 18" standard bib. Order from your dealer or call Tidi Brand at (800) 521-1314 for additional information on the bib.

Pearl 158

RetarDENT Toothpaste
by Rowpar Pharmaceuticals, Inc.

My long-time friend, Dr. Omer Reed, asked me to try his RetarDENT toothpaste. I have been using it with great results. A few years ago, a survey by the U.S. Army found that soldiers were motivated to care for their teeth, not for plaque control, but by the desire to be kissable! RetarDENT Toothpaste provides the "breath of confidence" to your patients and helps maintain oral wellness between visits to your office. This product and the companion RetarDEX Oral Rinse contain chlorine dioxide, which has the ability to break down the volatile sulfur compounds (VSC) that cause oral malodor. Rowpar's products have peer-reviewed, published research showing their safety and efficacy. Besides controlling bad breath, research has shown an 87 percent reduction in bleeding on probing and a 75 percent reduction if probing scores are 4 mm or more. Call Rowpar Pharmaceuticals, Inc. toll-free at (800) 643-3337 to place an order. The products are sold only to dental professionals and selected dental supply companies.

Chapter Eleven

Chairside Amenities and Patient Home Care

$\mathscr{P}earl$ *159*

Chainless Patient Bibs
by Crosstex

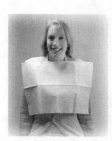

Here's a great idea from the people at Crosstex. If your office is anything like ours, you are constantly misplacing, throwing away, and, in general, losing those shiny chains with the alligator clips on the end that hold the patient bib in place. Crosstex solves that by placing adhesive tabs on the bib. Presto! Just remove the tabs, and you can quickly stick the bib to the patient's clothing for a simple, easy setup. The bibs come in two-ply and three-ply, with a plastic backing to protect the patient. They are available in a variety of colors in the standard 13" x 19" bib. We use them a lot for the quick patient appointments where minimal protection is necessary, such as new-patient exams, quick adjustment visits, and the like. Give Crosstex a call for more info at (800) 223-2497 or contact your dealer.

Pearl 160

The Comfy Wrap
by Comfy Concepts

I was walking through the Chicago Midwinter Meeting with Rhonda (my dental assistant and an assistant editor of DE) late in the afternoon. We had been on the exhibit floor all day looking for new products to try and were really dragging when we came upon the Comfy Concepts booth. As we stood in front of the booth, they draped a soft, lightweight, flexible wrap around our necks. The wrap was heated, and the warmth seemed to permeate and relax all the muscles of my neck and shoulders. It felt wonderful. The Comfy

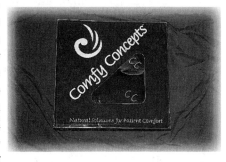

Wrap also has a small pocket in which you can place a choice of herbs that will give off a therapeutic aroma. I thought that if this could make me feel so good in the middle of an exhibit floor, just think how our patients would feel if we greeted them with a nice warm Comfy Wrap when they arrive at the office. This falls into the category of five-star service that will set our practices apart from the others. The Comfy Wrap addresses your patients' unspoken needs and shows your concern for their comfort and well-being. Comfy Concepts also has an Eye Pillow and a Lumbar Pillow for your patients' comfort needs. I think this is a great concept. Your patients will be touched in a simple, down-to-earth manner that they will feel and remember. They will love you for your thoughtfulness. Can they get this at the managed-care office down the street? Building a trust between you and your patients will help your practice grow and let your patients know how much you care. To order this great product, call Comfy Concepts at (888) 842-1277.

Pearl 161

NTI-TSS, Inc. Clenching-Suppression System
by Heraeus Kulzer

This device is for your patients who suffer from symptoms that can include frequent and recurring tension headaches, aching jaw muscles, and sore teeth. To use this technique, you must consider a redefinition of bruxism as severe clenching, with or without forcible lateral excursions. Therefore, the intensity of clenching dictates the severity of grinding.

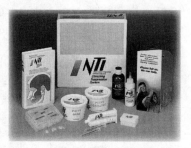

So, placing a "night guard" only compounds the problem, because the patient now clenches the appliance you placed and gets the same symptoms. The high-intensity contractions of these powerful muscles cause pain in the muscle and the surrounding tissues, joints, and muscles. If the intensity of the clenching could be reduced, the source of the pain could be effectively reduced.

The NTI-TSS, Inc. device is simple to fabricate in the office during a one-visit, 30-minute appointment with no impressions or lab fees. It is a simple device that fits on the upper centrals and has a plane that contacts the lower incisors and opens the bite so that no teeth can come together in centric or excursive movements. As the lower incisors sense moderate to severe pressure, a reflex response of the trigeminal signals the temporalis to relax, thereby reducing the clenching intensity. Pain is reduced or eliminated in just a few days.

Heraeus Kulzer has put together a complete kit, including patient information and a videotape describing the technique. It has been used successfully on thousands of patients who have experienced a reduction of symptoms. You can qualify which patients this device will help by using a simple examination and palpation of the temporalis muscle.

Order from NTI-TSS, Inc. at 1-877-4NTITSS; or visit their Web site at www.kulzer.com.

Pearl 162

The DentaPedic Pad
by DentaPedic Products

As I lecture around the country, there is always a lot of interest when I talk about this pad that will make any dental chair extremely comfortable. I am constantly asked about disinfecting the pad. DentaPedic products are covered with a PU Wetsafe impermeable material that will not absorb any liquid. The cover can be cleaned with the standard disinfectants that you use to clean your treatment rooms. The Swedish foam material responds to your body heat and then contours to relieve all pressure points. I have had the pads on my chairs for more than two years now, and my patients love them. 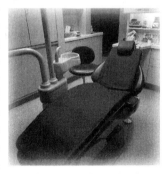 Most say they have never been that comfortable in a dental chair before. This is the same material that John Glenn said was so comfortable on his recent ride into space. This is a great way to show that you really care about your patients' comfort. Call DentaPedic Products at (800) 500-0518 to place your order or for more information. Ask for Dick Roach.

● ●

Pearl 163

Disposable Nitrous Hood
by Accutron

For you nitrous-oxide analgesia-users out there, this is a product that I have been using since it first came out a few years ago. Our patients love them because they know they are getting a new, clean hood at each visit, and they don't have to worry about who used it before they did. The hoods come in a variety of sizes and colors. The color signifies the scent that is associated with the hood. The patients really like the scent; it makes the experience much more comfortable. The hoods are readily adapted to scavenger systems and rubber goods. If you use nitrous oxide analgesia in your office, you owe it to yourself and your patients to try these hoods. This is just one more piece to the infection-control puzzle. Call Accutron about the Disposable Nitrous Hood or order from your dealer.

● ●

$\mathcal{P}earl\ 164$

Salix SST
by Scandinavian Naturals, Inc.

The uncomfortable feeling of dry mouth (xerostomia) affects millions of people, particularly the elderly. Now comes an all-new way of solving an old problem—Salix is natural relief. Dry mouth is one of the most common side effects associated with numerous medications, and it is a frequent side effect of people receiving chemotherapy. Dry mouth is not only irritating, but it also causes difficulties in speaking, swallowing, and eating, as well as an increased susceptibility to decay. Too often we, as dentists, do not have a solution, so people turn to hard candy or throat lozenges, which further damage the teeth. Salix is a simple, easy-to-use tablet that you allow to dissolve in the mouth. It tastes great and provides an instant, long-lasting effect. It is clinically proven not to cause decay. We keep a supply in our office to give to patients as starter samples, and we refer patients to pharmacies and health-food stores that carry the product. Call Scandinavian Naturals, Inc. at (800) 288-2844.

● ●

$\mathcal{P}earl\ 165$

FlossCard
by Oramaax Dental Products

For years, I have given my patients samples of dental floss from various manufacturers, and I paid for the privilege of handing out those floss samples with the manufacturer's ad on the package. With FlossCard, you can do something different—give away floss samples with your ad on the package. The FlossCard is a flat,

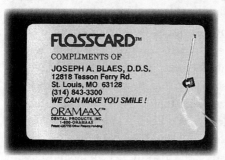

credit-card dispenser personalized with your message and filled with 12 yards of floss. The card goes into your patient's wallet or pocket and is there when he or she needs it. Since the FlossCard prominently features your name, address, and phone number, it is far superior to any floss you may currently be giving out to your patients. My patients really love the dispensers, and we usually give each patient two and ask him or her to give one to a friend. Call (800) ORAMAAX (672-6229) for a free sample.

$\mathscr{P}earl$ *166*

Encore Plus
by Fresh Concepts

I have used different air-freshening systems in the office and found them, in general, to be heavy and oppressive. Encore Plus is a metered aerosol air-refreshening system that is programmable. The system will tell you when to replace the fragrance and the batteries. The fragrances are great, not overpowering at all. Encore Plus is designed to utilize the positive effects of Aroma Therapy, with many different fragrances extracted from the oils of flowers, fruits, and organic plants. Its purpose is to help reduce stress and relax your patients with these pleasant fragrances. No more medicament smells when entering your office! They also have a WORLDWIND mini that is ideal for smaller offices. I am very pleased to have found this product and to recommend it to you. To order Encore Plus, call Fresh Concepts direct at (800) 537-3745.

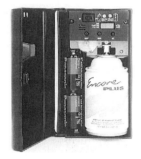

● ●

Pearl 167

All Clear
by Septodont

U npleasant odors don't have to be a part of your practice any-
more. The All Clear Molecular Adsorber attracts and eliminates
irritating and potentially harmful odors of fumes and gases to
help create a safer, more pleasant work environment. We started using

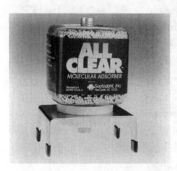 this little wonder in the sterilizing room to
control the odor of the chemiclave. It
worked so well that we put them in every
room in the office. Glutaraldehyde, darkroom chemicals, acrylic monomers, bonding chemicals—all these odors and more
are attracted by All Clear's magic pellets.
The pellets even change color to tell you
when to change them. Our patients have
commented on the lack of obnoxious odors
and have said that the office doesn't smell like a dental office. What a
great comment! The infection-control gurus recommend having one in
every treatment room. All Clear is a great product. Try it; you'll smell
better! Order from your dealer or call Septodont at (800) 872-8305.

$\mathcal{P}earl$ *168*

Mint Snuff All-Mint Chew
by Oregon Mint Snuff Company

It's baseball-fever time and the season is in full swing. What do you see a lot of the players doing? That's right, spitting and chewing! This habit is very much like playing Russian roulette. When I have a patient who has a smokeless-tobacco habit, I usually tell him or her all the horror stories about how many young people end up. Since most of us think we are immortal, especially when we are young, this does not have much of an impact. After all, if professional athletes do it, it must be OK. At the ADA meeting in Washington, DC, I came across a new use for the mint leaf that could very well save people's 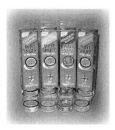 lives. Now I have an alternative to offer patients who chew and spit. I can encourage them to quit by using Mint Snuff All-Mint Chew and All-Mint Pouches, a healthy alternative that has none of the dangerous properties found in tobacco. But the can is identical to smokeless tobacco, and it looks the same...so the social part is the same. It contains no sugar, no salt, no tobacco, and no nicotine. The juices and the pulp can be eaten (no more spitting), and the mouth smells and feels fresh. The products were developed primarily as an aid for those wishing to get away from chewing tobacco. Over 12 million people use some form of smokeless tobacco, and the largest increase is among young people from ages eight to 17-years-old. Most of the youngsters are doing it because it is the "in" thing to do, but now you can offer them an alternative. Tobacco Intervention Network will provide you with free samples to distribute to the public. There is absolutely no cost to you. All you have to do is call (800) 938-1957 or visit www.quittobacco.com. So what are you waiting for? This tremendous service that you can offer to your community will not happen until you pick up the phone.

Pearl 169

Smile Gourmet
by Smile Sugarfree Candy, Inc.

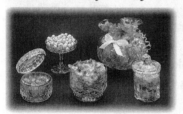

It's always the little things in life that provide the most pleasure. Take candy. I can remember riding my bike over to the corner grocery store and buying a nickel's worth of penny candy that would last all afternoon. But candy is sadly denied more and more as we grow older. Bad for our teeth. Bad for our waistlines. In such a sad world, a dentist, of all people, came to the rescue in 1990. Dr. Harry Harcsztark came upon a unique process that blends and cures fruit flavors, creating candy that is just as delicious as the candy we loved so much as children. He called his company Smile Sugarfree Candy and began selling to dentists whose patients loved candy, but whose teeth shouldn't be exposed. Then, doctors treating patients with diabetes were able to provide candy. As we try to set our dental practices apart, one unusual, but extremely well-received, program is a "thank you" gift of the world's best-tasting sugarfree candy, shipped to the patient in a wide variety of classy containers. This company offers gifts ranging from plastic "apples" to full-lead crystalware to Tiffany-brand quality gifts that show your office is a cut above the rest and that you care. We have been using this program for the reception room, as a welcome to the office, as thanks for referrals, to other referring doctors, to the health-food stores that refer to us, and for many other occasions. Great-tasting, sugarfree hard candies, lollipops, jellybeans, caramels, and chocolate balls, shipped in a wide variety of gift packaging—along with a personalized note from your office—provide the extra touch that makes your office the "Ritz-Carlton" of personalized dental services. Give this company a call at (800) SMILE-14, fax to (201) 991-8229 or e-mail smile@sugarfree.com to order or to obtain more information. Your patients will love this one!

Pearl 170

Blue's Clues
by Oral-B

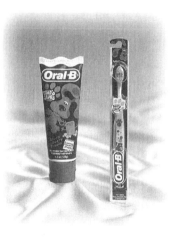

If the reaction of my grandchildren is any indication, Oral-B has a hit with the Blue's Clues toothbrushes and toothpaste. The grandkids went crazy over them! That makes brushing the children's teeth less of a hassle. Each Oral-B Blue's Clues toothbrush features the show's main character, Blue, with one of her friends. It comes in 16 different variations and is especially designed to fit the hand and mouth of young preschoolers, which helps them learn how to brush. The Oral-B Berry Bubble toothpaste squeezes out in a bright blue gel with a paw-print shape. Contact your Oral-B rep for more information.

$\mathcal{P}earl$ 171

SmartBrush
by The SmartBrush Corporation

I came across this brush at the ADA meeting in San Francisco and have been using it myself since then. This is a brush designed by a dentist whose patients had difficulty brushing those hard-to-reach tooth and gum surfaces of the mouth. It is unlike any brush you have ever seen in that you can rotate the head 45 degrees in either direction, and you can change the shape of the bristles by bending the head. I know this all sounds kind of crazy and gimmicky, but it really works. This is one of those things that you have to try yourself, so give SmartBrush Corporation a call toll-free at (877) 476-2782 or fax them at (770) 381-9038 and ask for a sample. I think you will like it as much as I do. Smart-Brush is being marketed only through dental offices and is not available in retail stores.

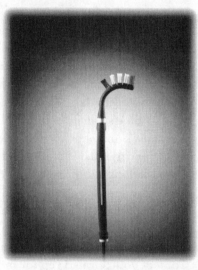

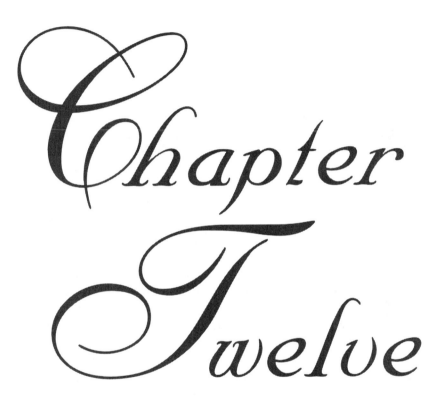

Chapter Twelve

Services

● ●

Pearl 172

The Seltzer Institute

I suspect that there are a lot of dentists out there like me. I am totally confused about how to make sense out of the high-tech dental market. Where do you go to get good information? If you go to the exhibit floor of most meetings, all you get is a lot of hype and promises and high-pressure sales techniques. When does it make sense to buy another computer, and what should you expect that computer to do, given today's advances in electronics? Have you bought an intraoral video camera, but find that it gathers more dust than pictures of teeth? If so, you are not alone! The untimely and unwise purchasing of high-tech equipment is one of the leading causes of financial difficulty, staff turmoil, and major personal frustration in many dental practices all over the country. What you need is not more equipment—or less equipment—but a better understanding of how to use the high-tech gear you already have and how to develop a strategy to buy equipment that makes sense for your office. Is there anyone out there who can give us an unbiased view of high-tech equipment? Yes. Steven M. Seltzer shares technology secrets unavailable anywhere else in dentistry. Steve is a nationally recognized expert on dental technology and what it can and cannot do for your practice. He speaks at meetings around the country, and I would recommend that you hear him. He also is available for consultation. Contact him at the Seltzer Institute at (800) 229-8967.

● ● ● ● ● ●

Pearl 173

Standard Operating Procedures (SOP) for Dentists
by Marsha Freeman

How many of you have always thought that it would be great to have a manual in the office with all of your procedures in it? What a great way to train a new staff member! But most of us have been too busy to create it. Well, now there is a book that will make it easy for you. Marsha will take you step by step through a model procedural manual that will help you develop your own in-house, customized procedural manual in much less time than you could create your own. A manual will create measurable standards for your practice. It also comes on a computer disk, and it has a money-back guarantee. How can you lose? Call Marsha at (800) 563-1454 and get organized!

$\mathcal{P}earl$ 174

"Dentists: An Endangered Species"
"Isn't It Wonderful When Patients Say 'Yes'"
by Dr. Paul Homoly

If you have been a reader for any length of time, you know that I do not recommend many books. I was on a long flight to Portland, Oregon, this summer and read what I consider to be a "must-read" for dentists who want a practice model that will allow them to survive and thrive in dentistry. I have heard Dr. Paul Homoly speak and know that his technical expertise and his marketing skills always were way ahead of the pack. I always have believed in the value of relationship-building in my practice. In his books, Dr. Homoly writes that the greatest values in dentistry are found within relationships, not restorations. These are books for doctor and staff. In the case of each one, you can buy just the book or you can take advantage of what I consider to be a great package offer. The package includes the book; a studio-produced, three-hour audio program that reinforces the book and includes staff training; and a computer disk that contains all the forms that you will need to get going. You can order this series from PennWell Books at (800) 752-9764. Don't miss this opportunity to move your practice to the next level!

• •

Pearl 175

"Patient Management: The Relationship Factor"
by Dr. Marvin Mansky

Marvin is a good friend of mine whom I met through the American Academy of Dental Practice Administration. At our annual meeting last year, Dr. Mansky presented a program that basically explained how to build relationships with our patients. He has edited a tape of that program to provide us all with some wonderful ideas and techniques. Marvin believes that understanding patient and dentist behavior is one of the most significant factors in building a successful and personally rewarding practice. In this program, he presents a number of concepts such as a five-minute anxiety cure for patients (or for anyone), how to be fully present without distraction for our patients, and how to be connected with our patients. He is able to simplify and improve the very complex interactions of the dentist/patient interchange. It is his belief that the mastery of simple, easy-to-learn techniques can significantly benefit the dentist interested in building a strong, private fee-for-service practice. This is an extremely practical tape that will enable you to form better relationships with everyone you meet. Call Dr. Mansky at (888) 808-8997 to order.

● ●

$\mathcal{P}earl$ 176

Magical Customer Service and the Statementless Professional Practice
by Patrick Wahl, DMD, MBA, and Lorraine Hollett

I do not often review an audiotape series in "Pearls," but this one is different. Dr. Pat Wahl and Lorraine Hollett have packed this tape series with vital information that you need to know. This is a complete system for collecting your fees at the time of service. Pat and Lorraine have drawn up a plan for you to follow that is foolproof. They will tell you how to stop lending patients your money by showing you how to find alternative financing for your patients. They hold your hand and take you step by step through their wonderful program of achieving zero accounts receivable. There is a large amount of printed material

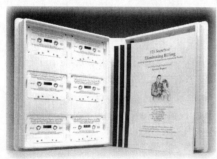

that includes scripts for you and your staff, the forms you will need, and answers to all of your objections about why this won't work in your practice. In addition, they will tell you how to wow your patients with "Knock Your Socks Off" customer service...how to make your practice stand out from the other practices

in your community. This is one of the keys to growing your fee-for-service practice. Call Office Magic Productions at (800) 750-8779 or visit their Web site at www.office magic.com.

$\mathscr{P}earl$ 177

Look, Mom...No Cavities!
How To Raise a Cavity-Free Child
by Gregory F. George, DDS

This is an excellent guide for today's concerned parent, packed with vital facts, techniques, and tips on preventing cavities in their children's teeth. Parents can discover everything they need to know and have a handy guide to answer future questions. Dr. George is a pediatric dentist in Buffalo, N.Y., who has dedicated his career to teaching patients to be cavity-free. Look Mom... No Cavities! is also available on an excellent videotape produced by Greg and on an audio-cassette tape, both of which are perfect companions to the book. To order, call PDC Press at (888) 292-1991 or call your local Patterson dealer. Check out the web site www.lookmom.com. Don't miss this one! If you are treating children in your practice, you cannot be without this book!

$\mathcal{P}earl$ 178

FluoriCheck Water Analysis Service
by Omnii Products

O mnii has introduced the first nationally available, doctor-dispensed fluoride test for determining the fluoride levels in homes. Fluoride supplements no longer can be prescribed based on the broad assumption that the parts per million (ppm) fluo-

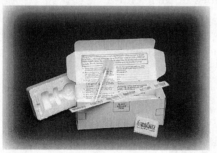

ride levels of communal or private water supplies are consistent. Well location and depth, surface water source, water system age, and in-home water filters all can lead to varying ppm levels within the same community. There are currently no fluoride-content, food-labeling requirements for any foods or beverages, including bottled water. Dentifrices marketed to children may be increasing the level of unintentional ingestion of therapeutic fluoride levels. All of these factors have been attributed to an increase in the incidence of fluorosis nationwide. Establishing the most important baseline—the ppm fluoride content of a child's primary drinking water source—can better control this. Until now, the availability of testing services to determine fluoride ppm levels in drinking water has been limited, unpredictable, and inconvenient. The FluoriCheck Water Analysis service eliminates these problems. Easy-to-follow instructions ensure quick and accurate results. Call Omnii Products at (800) 445-3386 to order or for more information. This could be a great practice-builder!

$\mathcal{P}earl$ *179*

Drug Information Handbook for Dentistry
by Lexi-Comp

I heard Dr. Harold L. Crossley speak at the Tennessee State Meeting in Nashville, and you need to get this book at once. Better yet, get it on CD-ROM and you can enhance the practice-management system that you are using with a system that will provide a patient-specific drug analysis. No office should be without this guide. It was designed and written by dentists for all dental professionals. It has more than 22 key points of information for each drug, including: use, usual dosage, effects on dental treatment, local anesthetic and vasoconstrictor precautions, and important drug interactions. You will get much more information from this important guide than you ever got when you called the physician's office of a medically compromised patient. Don't wait; order yours today! Ask for Lexi-Comp's Academic Dental Software package on CD-ROM by calling (800) 837-5394.

● ●

Pearl 180

The ASDC Kid's Mouth Book
by Dr. Theodore P. Croll

My good friend, Dr. Ted Croll, sent me the recently published second edition of this great book. The first edition was published in 1993, and it has become the recommended source for parents, kids, pediatricians, school nurses, and anyone else interested in children's dentistry. Many dentists have bought multiple copies for their own reception rooms and as gifts for local school libraries, colleagues' offices, or local pediatricians' offices. Ted has donated all of his royalties from this project to the American Society of Dentistry for Children (ASDC).

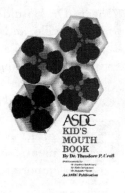

Every dental office should have a copy of the Kid's Mouth Book in the reception room. To place your order or for additional information, call the ASDC at (800) 637-2732 today.

$\mathcal{P}earl$ *181*

Smile After Smile II
by High Impact Marketing

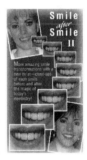

D r. Tom Hughes has done it again with another fantastic video that features the smile transformations of real patients right before your eyes. This is even better than his first video, because now you will see close-ups of each smile—both before and after treatment. Now viewers can clearly see the miraculous difference that modern dental techniques can make in their smiles and in their lives. This is life changing!!! Smile After Smile II is set to soothing music and runs continuously for two hours. It will provide a fascinating and eye-opening experience for your patients, who are guaranteed to ask questions like, "What can you do for my smile?" Don't wait; order yours now! Tom has made a special offer to the readers of *Dental Equipment & Materials*. Call High Impact Marketing at (719) 488-0808 to order yours.

Index

C

Calibra, 143

Cameras, 15-18

Carbide lab burs, 158

Cements, 135-147:
RecyXVLC (Vitremer Luting Cement), 136-137; Fuji Plus capsules, 137; PermaCem, 138; Rely X ARC adhesive resin cement, 139; Panavia 21, 140; Compolute Aplicap, 141; Nexus Universal Luting System, 142; Nexus 2 Luting System, 142; Calibra, 143; Operatory Kit, 143; Encore Solo, 144; ProxiDiscs, 144; Provilink, 145; TempBond™ Clear, 146; True-Grip tips, 147

Chainless patient bibs, 178

Chairside amenities and patient home care, 177-190: chainless patient bibs, 178; Comfy Wrap, 179; Eye Pillow, 179; Lumbar Pillow, 179; NTI-TSS, Inc. clenching-suppression system, 180-181; DentaPedic pad, 181; PU Wetsafe, 181; disposable nitrous hood, 182; Salix SST, 183; FlossCard, 184;

Encore Plus, 185; WORLDWIND, 185; All Clear, 186; Mint Snuff All-Mint Chew, 187; Smile Gourmet, 188; Blue's Clues, 189; Oral-B Berry Bubble toothpaste, 189; SmartBrush, 190

Chemiclave sterilizer, 30

Chlorhexi Prep, 97

C-LECT crown, 101

Clenching-suppression system, 180-181

Color Check, 19

Comfy Wrap, 179

Compolute Aplicap, 141

Composi-Tight, 78

Cosmetic/esthetic dentistry. SEE Restorative, cosmetic/ esthetic dentistry.

Craniometer, The, 37

Crown and bridge restorative, 99-119:
Block inlay bridge, 100; C-LECT crown, 101; Procera, 102; IPS Empress2, 103; dental button, 104; Luxatemp Automix Plus system, 105-106; E-Z Temp inlay and E-Z Temp onlay, 106-107; flexible clearance tabs, 107; EZ contact, 108;

G

Gendex GX-LC, 31

Gloves, 6-8

Gluma® Desensitizer, 59

G-ring, 78

Great White Gold Series burs, 111

GYRO air-bearing handpiece, 24

H

Handpieces, 24, 26-28

Heliomolar® Flow, 77

Highlight view light, 81

Home care.
   SEE Chairside amenities and patient home care.

I

IBC Brush, 2

Implant-Prophy+, 164

Impressions, 121-133:
   Imprint II, 122-123;
   Take 1, 123;
   Position Penta impression material, 124;
   Imprint II Quick Step HB/LB impression material, 125;
   Imprint II SBR occlusal registration material, 126;
   Easy Tray, 127-128;
   Easy Base, 128;
   SureLoc, 128;
   Clinician's Choice quad impression tray, 129;
   three-way trays, 130;
   Kromopan 100, 131;
   Alginator, 132;
   Jumbo syringe system, 133

Imprint II, 122-123

Imprint II Quick Step HB/LB impression material, 125

Imprint II SBR occlusal registration material, 126

Instruments, 33-42:
   DuraLite instruments, 34;
   Zekrya gingival retractor and protector, 35;
   SuperMat Retainerless Matrix System, 36;
   The Craniometer, 37;
   Tri Auto-ZX, 38;
   Endo Analyzer 8005, 39;
   XCP film holder, 40;
   Profin Directional System, 41; Expandex, 42.
   SEE ALSO
   Materials, equipment, and supplies.

IntegraPost Carrier, 91

IntegraPost System, 91

Intraoral camera mirror attachment, 18;
LH systems cleaners, 19;
Fixscent, 19;
Color Check, 19;
TTL telescopes, 20;
Zeon illuminator, 21, 23;
Pearls, 22;
Bora high-speed handpiece, 24;
GYRO air-bearing handpiece, 24;
prismatic loupes, 25;
KaVo 640B handpiece, 26-27;
KaVO 642B handpiece, 26-27;
430 Series high-speed handpieces, 27;
electric micromotor handpiece, 28;
RotoMix, 29;
Chemiclave sterilizer, 30;
Gendex GX-LC, 31;
EzeeKleen 2.5, 32.
SEE ALSO
Instruments.

Matrix systems for composites, 79-80

Microbrush, 3

MicroDose, 97

Mint Snuff All-Mint Chew, 187

Mr. Bond, 153

Multi-colloid technique, 159-160

Multi-Cup Dentures, 152

Nanofillers, 54

Nexus 2 Luting System, 142

Nexus Universal Luting System, 142

Nifty Strip, 94

Nonlatex dental dam, 11

NTI-TSS, Inc. clenching-suppression system, 180-181

Nu Source International, 19

OneGloss, 85

Opalescence tooth whitening family, 171:
Opalescence F, 171;
Opalescence Quick, 171;
Opalescence Xtra, 171

Operatory Kit, 143

OptiBond Solo Plus™, 55

OptiBond Solo, 53

Optilux 501, The, 80

Optipost System, 93

Oral-B Berry Bubble toothpaste, 189

OralCDx®, 14

Osteo Graf/LD, 88-89

S

Safety-wipes, 5

Salix SST, 183

Seal & Protect™, 58-59

Sealants.
   SEE Prophy, sealants.

Seltzer Institute, 192

Services, 191-201:
   Seltzer Institute, 192;
   Standard Operating
   Procedures (SOP) for
   Dentists, 193;
   Dentists: An Endangered
   Species. "Isn't It Wonderful
   When Patients Say 'Yes'",
   194;
   Patient Management: The
   Relationship Factor, 195;
   Magical Customer Service
   and the Statementless
   Professional Practice, 196;
   "Look, Mom…No
   Cavities!" How to Raise a
   Cavity-Free Child, 197;
   FluoriCheck Water Analysis
   service, 198;
   Drug Information
   Handbook for Dentistry,
   199;
   The ASDC Kid's
   Mouth Book, 200;
   Smile After Smile II, 201

SG-Cutter Blade, 158

Sharpness testing device, 44

Shock 'ta' Clear, 13

Shorter-Than-Short and new
   finishing strips, 113

Single-dose needle tubes, 73

Single-patient applicators, 97

SmartBrush, 190

Smile After Smile II, 201

Smile Catalog, The, 62

Smile Gourmet, 188

Snap-Stone, 114

Snoop caries detecting dye, 96

Sof-Tray Sheets, 171

Soft Relining System, 155

SoftLine, 154

Stabident, 47

Standard Operating
   Procedures (SOP)
   for Dentists, 193

Sterilizer, 30

Steri-Tip, 10

Stop-Strip, 79

Strip-Aid, 79

SuperBuff, 85

SuperMat retainerless
   matrix system, 36

Supplies and equipment.
   SEE Materials, equipment,
   and supplies.

SureFil, 70

SureLoc, 128

Symmetry Facial Plane
   Relator, 65

Syringe covers, 52

X

Y

Z